DIAGNOSTIC SKILLS IN CLINICAL LABORATORY SCIENCE

DIAGNOSTIC SKILLS IN CLINICAL LABORATORY SCIENCE

▶ **Connie R. Mahon, MS, CLS, MT(ASCP)**

Director, Clinical Laboratory Officers Course
Clinical Laboratory Science Program
Walter Reed Army Medical Center
Adjunct Assistant Professor of Pathology
George Washington University
School of Medicine and Health Sciences
Washington, DC

▶ **David G. Fowler, PhD, CLS(NCA)**

Professor and Chair
Department of Clinical Laboratory Sciences
University of Mississippi Medical Center
Jackson, Mississippi

McGRAW-HILL

Medical Publishing Division

New York / Chicago / San Francisco / Lisbon / London / Madrid / Mexico City
Milan / New Delhi / San Juan / Seoul / Singapore / Sydney / Toronto

The McGraw·Hill Companies

Diagnostic Skills in Clinical Laboratory Science

1 2 3 4 5 6 7 8 9 0   DOC/DOC   0 9 8 7 6 5 4 3

ISBN 0-07-136120-0

This book was set in New Aster by Deirdre Sheean of McGraw-Hill Professional's Hightstown, NJ composition unit.
The editors were Michael Brown and Janene Matragrano Oransky.
The production supervisor was Catherine Saggese.
The designer was Marsha Cohen/Parallelogram.
The cover designer was Elizabeth Pisacreta.
The index was prepared by Andover Publishing Services.
RR Donnelley was printer and binder.

This book is printed on acid-free paper.

Library of Congress Cataloging-in-Publication Data

Mahon, Connie R.
    Diagonostic skills in clinical laboratory science / Connie R. Mahon, David G. Fowler.
       p. ; cm..
    Includes bibliographical references.
    ISBN 0-07-136120-0 (alk. paper)
    1. Diagnosis, Laboratory—Case studies.   2. Medical laboratory technology—Case studies.
  I. Fowler, David G.   II. Title.
    [DNLM: 1. Clinical Laboratory Techniques—methods—Problems and Exercises.   2.
    Laboratory Techniques and Procedures—Problems and Excercises. QY 18.2 M216d 2003]
    RB37.5.M247   2003
  616.07'56—dc21

                          2003042057

▶ CONTENTS

Appendix A

ANTIGEN-ANTIBODY CHARACTERISTIC CHART AND

TABLES OF REFERENCE RANGES

Appendix B

ANSWERS TO LEARNING ACTIVITIES AND CASE SUMMARIES

Roberta Banks

► ACKNOWLEDGMENTS

We are grateful to the contributing authors and to many other individuals who have made significant suggestions and invaluable comments on ways to develop this project. Many thanks to former students Melissa Nedry, Matt Rubinstein, CPT Steven Craig, and CPT Jason Cortey, colleagues Bill Turcan and Lynn Ingram, and Dr. Dan Cruser for reviewing the hematology cases and providing helpful comments. Our appreciation also goes to Diana Mass and Steven Zollo for their encouragement and support.

► PREFACE

Use of the case-based approach is not a novel way to enhance critical thinking skills. In this method of learning, the student identifies certain critical facts and applies basic information previously learned to resolve a given problem. A student tends to develop a better understanding of the clinical situation by identifying the situation and actively finding a solution. So, what is different about *Diagnostic Skills in Clinical Laboratory Science* from other texts that use case studies to promote problem-solving skills?

Diagnostic Skills in Clinical Laboratory Science is the combination of a workbook and CD-ROM that shows the student how to resolve a problem in a given situation. The student works on each case using both components. Similar to a building-block approach to learning, this method gives the student learning assessment activities that progress from the identification of pertinent patient clinical information to the correlation of laboratory tests relevant to the patient's initial diagnosis, and ultimately to the resolution of a laboratory test discrepancy. The student is able to work on cases that may require a simple identification of the etiologic agent of an infectious disease or a determination of the cause of a blood incompatibility.

The student, an active participant in his or her learning experience, is guided through the maize of gathering and interpreting data and of problem identification. While working on each case, the student is asked to obtain the patient's laboratory tests results from the simulated laboratory information system (LIS) contained in the CD-ROM. He or she records the results in the laboratory report forms included in the workbook.

It is our belief that when the student reviews the laboratory data in the LIS and manually transfers the laboratory results to the report forms in the workbook, he or she becomes more actively involved in the learning process. The navigation of the program in the CD-ROM is user-friendly and is designed so that the user may access the laboratory results when needed.

The cases are varied in their level of difficulty and complexity but represent the disease conditions usually encountered in the clinical laboratory setting. Most of the cases also require integration of laboratory results from more than one clinical discipline, making the cases multidisciplinary. The student, for example, is exposed to data, such as hematology or chemistry laboratory findings, which is important in determining the significance of a bacterial isolate.

Our intent is to stimulate the student's thought process to form ideas, relearn basic concepts, and apply previously developed skills. We hope that by working on the case studies, both students and faculty will find the exchange of thoughts and ideas enjoyable and be encouraged to further investigation concerning the case by reading recommended reference materials. Finally, we find *Diagnostic Skills in Clinical Laboratory Science* an appropriate learning tool for students of other health care professions including nurses and physician assistants. We also hope that the user finds working on the cases a rewarding adventure.

Connie R. Mahon
David G. Fowler

▶ INTRODUCTION

With the evolution of health care over the past several years, it has become necessary for the clinical laboratory practitioner to take more control in the practice of clinical laboratory science. Clinical laboratory practitioners must be able to provide the level of expertise that is required for effective patient care management in the managed-care arena. They must also become more responsible for the outcomes of clinical laboratory testing. Therefore, clinical laboratory practitioners must develop a logical system for investigating problems or discrepancies that may be encountered in clinical practice. It is important for them to be able to define the problem, identify indicators, and analyze and synthesize data. They must also be able to reason out the steps they take in the problem-resolution and decision-making processes.

Hence, the focus in Clinical Laboratory Science (CLS) education must move from the traditional analytical phase of testing to a much broader scope of practice, with a focus on the preanalytical and postanalytical phases. As CLS students, you must enhance your problem-solving and critical-thinking skills. You must become skilled in gathering and analyzing the information that is essential for solving problems or resolving discrepancies.

To help prepare you for your new role, we developed the student workbook and CD-ROM *Diagnostic Skills in Clinical Laboratory Science*. This learning tool uses a case-based approach and is aimed at stimulating your thinking processes. The workbook and CD-ROM combination is intended to provide you with a mechanism that will help you use previously learned skills while working through patient cases. Each case provides an opportunity for you to develop clinical reasoning skills.

What Is Case-Based Learning?

Case-based or problem-based learning is a method of enhancing your critical-thinking skills by enabling you to actively participate in the learning process. In problem-based learning, you develop a better understanding of the given situation by effectively identifying the facts and information that are necessary for dealing with the situation. Problem-based learning enables you to integrate knowledge from many disciplines in order to solve problems of the type that you may encounter in clinical practice.

With this approach, you are given problems in the form of cases. You are directed to identify the problem or determine whether a discrepancy exists. You are then to find the solution to the problem or the resolution of the discrepancy by going through a critical-thinking process: interpreting laboratory test results, using identification schemas, and relating the results to the patient's clinical presentation. By doing this, you develop the ability to reason out diagnostic and identification decisions.

Goals and Objectives

The goal of the *Diagnostic Skills in Clinical Laboratory Science* workbook and CD-ROM is to enhance and assess your problem-solving and decision-making skills in clinical disciplines. On completion of the learning assessment activities given for each case, you will be able to

- Identify pertinent information regarding the patient's clinical presentation and determine the relevance of the laboratory tests requested on this patient.
- Apply previously acquired knowledge and skills to interpret laboratory results.
- Interpret laboratory data and correlate the information with the situation presented.
- Describe possible patient outcomes.
- Obtain appropriate feedback on your resolution of the problem.

Instructions

As a user of the *Diagnostic Skills in Clinical Laboratory Science* workbook and CD-ROM program, you will find that you are being asked to take on a new role. Whereas with many other CD-ROM programs or workbooks, you were a passive recipient of information, here you are given the opportunity to become an active participant in your own learning experience.

We have chosen cases that represent a variety of the disease conditions that you are most likely to encounter in your clinical laboratory setting. Working through each patient's problems gives you the opportunity to integrate a wide variety of information that you have previously learned. Try not to focus too much on simply getting the "right answer," although this is important. Instead, use this learning tool to stimulate your thought processes, formulate ideas, and review concepts that you may have forgotten or not fully understood. Hopefully, working on the patient cases will encourage you to further reading of the recommended texts and references as well as articles in the current scientific literature that your instructor may assign.

Components and Format of the Learning Tool

The learning activities in *Diagnostic Skills in Clinical Laboratory Science* have two components: a workbook and a simulated laboratory information system (LIS) in a CD-ROM format. You will need both components to work on each patient's case.

The workbook is designed to provide you with a system for exploring patients' problems and disease states. The process is very dynamic, as you must look for signs and indicators and analyze the available data. You may be asked to apply deductive reasoning to the problem or discrepancy you have identified and to describe how you will attempt to solve the problem or resolve the discrepancy.

The learning activities provided by the workbook include

Patient clinical history and progress reports. In the workbook, you will find a
simulated patient medical record that provides you with the patient's clinical history, the admitting diagnosis, the clinician's notes and course of
action, and notes on the patient's progress.

Laboratory reports. There are laboratory report forms for chemistry, hematology, and microbiology in the workbook on which you are to record laboratory test results. You access the patient's test results from the LIS in the CD-
ROM.

Laboratory worksheets. The workbook presents you with worksheets for antibody
identification panel on which you may record your results and identify the
antibody(ies) that may be involved in the case.

Learning assessment questions and study guide. You will find study questions
that assess your ability to correlate laboratory results with disease states,
interpret critical values, and resolve discrepancies. You may ask your
instructor to provide you with feedback on your responses, or you may
review your own work by referring to the recommended readings and
references.

Because you will be asked to work back and forth between the workbook and
the CD-ROM, it is important that you follow closely the instructions provided
in the workbook. The learning activities in the workbook direct you when to
use the CD-ROM and guide you in resolving the case with questions related
to data collection, interpretation, and correlation.

The CD-ROM provides you with

Patient history and demographic data. You will be given information on the
patient that will help you establish the case.

Simulated laboratory information system. You will access the simulated LIS
to obtain patient results and other data that may be required to resolve the
case. The navigation of the program in the CD-ROM is user-friendly and
intuitive, with drop-down menus and well-designed buttons. The lab data
are not presented as part of the case history but are available to you when
you request them. The computer program in the CD-ROM is designed so
that you can access each case independently and exit and reenter the program before completion of the case.

Format of the Patient Cases

PATIENT INFORMATION AND PROGRESS REPORTS

The simulated patient record contains the patient's name and identification
number (ID). You will need the patient's name and ID to obtain the patient's
lab results in the LIS. The patient's admission information, such as physical

exam findings, admission diagnosis, and primary complaints, is included, along with demographic data. The patient history is given as clinician's notes. Then the course of action or treatment plan is given. This is followed by reports on the patient's progress and ultimate outcome. The cases vary in length and complexity, and in the degree of detail presented.

LEARNING ACTIVITIES

The pages that follow the patient records give the learning activities. For each case, you are presented with learning issues; learning issues are similar to objectives, to help you achieve the goal stated for the learning activity. You will be asked to respond in writing to specific questions and to provide explanations or a rationale for your responses. The questions in the first part of the learning activity involve data gathering. You will be asked to record laboratory test results on the worksheets provided in the workbook. You may also be asked to provide a rationale for the clinician's course of action or treatment plan; you should write down your ideas, hunches, or hypotheses. Your learning will be directly proportional to the effort you invest in thinking about the problems and your responses to the study questions.

How to Use the Workbook and CD-ROM Combination

Use the cases provided in the workbook and the information contained in the CD-ROM to motivate your own inquiry strategy. At each step, you will have an opportunity to compare your responses with the responses provided in the workbook or to request feedback from your instructor. A review of the specific topic and the disease state or conditions related to the cases presented in the workbook is available on the CD-ROM.

Follow these basic steps in using the workbook and CD-ROM:

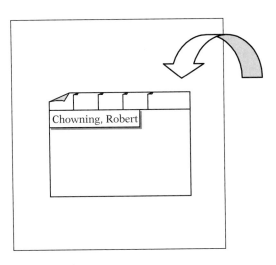

1. Select a patient. Patients are arranged alphabetically.

Chowning, Robert

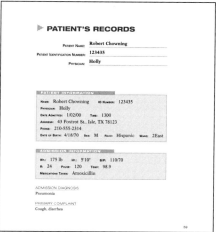

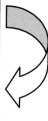

2. Read the patient information and progress reports in the patient's medical record.

3. Follow the instructions outlined in the Learning Activities section. Respond to the questions pertaining to the information presented.

4. Record laboratory data on work-sheet.

5. Access the CD-ROM for information when you are directed to do so. The CD-ROM will provide you with instructions on how to navigate the program.

Who Can Use This Learning Tool?

This workbook/CD-ROM combination is designed primarily for CLS/MT students who have completed didactic courses in at least one clinical discipline. The students may have completed the clinical practicum or may be preparing for their clinical rotations at the affiliate sites. It can also be used by students and professionals in other health sciences (e.g., physician assistants or nurses) who are interested in learning how to apply their knowledge to real-life situations and are looking to integrate laboratory findings from different disciplines and apply them to a particular patient condition.

It is also designed for clinical laboratory science educators and other health science faculty who would like to incorporate case-based learning materials into their students' coursework. These materials may serve as an adjunct to stimulate and integrate the students' learning. CLS faculty who have developed expertise in one clinical discipline may find these materials valuable in strengthening and expanding their ability to integrate two or more clinical disciplines from the perspective of teaching a disease state or condition.

Important Considerations for Instructors

This workbook and CD-ROM are designed to be used by a single individual, although working in small groups and learning from one another is encouraged and could also be fun. Faculty may choose to assign students specific cases to work individually or allow the students to work in small groups. In small-group discussions, one member of the group may be designated as the facilitator, or the faculty may serve in this role. The primary responsibilities of the facilitator are to monitor the group's discussions and progress and to guide the exchanges of ideas.

In traditional problem-based learning (PBL), students are directed to formulate their learning issues. In this program, we have developed the learning issues that in traditional PBL would have been determined by the students, either as assigned work or during group interactions. Thus, the information provided here is only an illustration of what students may find out and learn on their own as they engage in case-based learning activities. While preparing this learning tool, the problem we encountered as authors was how to intercede and facilitate in printed form. The flexibility of small-group discussions in traditional PBL is given up, but it can be recaptured by both students and faculty. We therefore wrote study questions only as a guide to direct learning toward a particular path.

Tips for Facilitators

Your main task as a facilitator is to assist in the group discussion by allowing members of the group to explore their own ideas. We strongly recommend that referring to the responses we provided be delayed to encourage self-directed learning by the students. As an instructor or facilitator, you may find our responses helpful in orienting yourself to the case. The following are suggestions that we thought might help you in guiding, directing, and if necessary mediating your students' discussions.

- Engage students in critical thinking by asking open-ended questions and exploring their responses.

- Provide straightforward but encouraging feedback about the performance of individuals and of the group as a whole.

- Monitor the group discussions by being an active participant and resource person without intervening or disrupting the group's activities. Provide information to get the group past a particular barrier when asked to do so, but do so thoughtfully.

- Encourage students to use and explore the wide variety of information resources available to them (other than yourself).

- Promote integration and further application of information by asking questions in addition to those listed in the workbook. Create a new or different "twist" to the case or patient outcome by changing the lab results or the treatment provided by the clinician. Encourage students to apply newly acquired information to other types of clinical situation.

- Finally, try to be flexible. Because some of the cases are multidisciplinary, they may include elements that are outside your areas of expertise. If this occurs, take the opportunity to learn and establish your own inquiry strategy. Even if you do not have enough experience in a particular area, you should still be able to ask critical questions.

Critical Points to Remember in Using This Learning Tool

- The *Diagnostic Skills in Clinical Laboratory Science* workbook and CD-ROM learning tool is not designed to serve as a textbook, providing comprehensive information on the topics presented. Rather, it is meant to introduce you to the process of integrating previously learned knowledge and applying it to clinical practice.

- Each case represents a certain condition or situation. It is meant to arouse your inquisitiveness about topics related to the particular condition or situation, to lead you to pursue the issues further, or to encourage you to formulate your own learning issues.

- The learning activities require you to write out your answers and transfer information from the CD-ROM to the workbook. The purpose of this activity is to enhance your learning through these motor activities and to create a written record of your thought processes that can be used for assessment or review.

- We suggest that you make your own list of topics that you would like to investigate further. Your instructor may also assign related topics or additional learning issues or points to consider.

- Finally, discovery is fun.

► BIBLIOGRAPHY AND RECOMMENDED READING

Forbes B, Sahm D, Weissfeld A: *Bailey and Scott's Diagnostic Microbiology,* 8th ed. St. Louis, Mosby, 2002.

Bishop M, Duben-Engelkirk, S, Fody E: *Clinical Chemistry: Principles & Procedures Correlations,* 4th ed. Philadelphia, Lippincott, 2000.

Carr J, Rodak B: *Clinical Hematology Atlas.* Philadelphia, Saunders, 1998.

Harmening D: *Modern Banking and Transfusion Practices,* 4th ed. Philadelphia, F. A. Davis, 1999.

Harmening D: *Clinical Hematology and Fundamentals of Hemostasis,* 3rd ed. Philadelphia, F. A. Davis, 1997.

Howard B et al: *Clinical and Pathogenic Microbiology,* 2nd ed. St. Louis, Mosby, 1994.

Koneman E et al: *Color Atlas and Textbook of Diagnostic Microbiology,* 5th ed. Philadelphia, Lippincott, l997.

Mahon CR, Manuselis G: *Textbook of Diagnostic Microbiology,* 2nd ed. Philadelphia, Saunders, 2000.

McKenzie SB: *Clinical Laboratory Hematology.* Upper Saddle River, NJ, Prentice-Hall, 2003.

Murray P, Baron EJ, Pfaller MA: *Manual of Clinical Microbiology,* 7th ed. Washington, DC, American Society for Microbiology, 2000.

Rodak B: *Hematology: Clinical Principles and Applications,* 2nd ed. Philadelphia, Elsevier, 2002.

Ryan K, Ray C: *Sherris Medical Microbiology, 4th ed.* New York: McGraw-Hill, 2004.

Strassinger S, DiLorenzo M: *Urinalysis and Body Fluids,* 4th ed. Philadelphia, F. A. Davis, 2001.

► PATIENT'S RECORDS

PATIENT NAME: **Roberta Banks**

PATIENT IDENTIFICATION NUMBER: **371440**

PHYSICIAN: **McCarthy**

PATIENT INFORMATION

NAME: Roberta Banks   ID NUMBER: 371440

PHYSICIAN: McCarthy

DATE ADMITTED: 11/30/02   TIME: 0940

ADDRESS: 499 Slaughter Lane, Someplace, MD 20202

PHONE: 000-533-4455

DATE OF BIRTH: 10/5/49   SEX: F   RACE: W

ADMISSION INFORMATION

WT.: 150 lb   HT.: 5'10"   B/P: 158/94

R: 17   PULSE: 83   TEMP.: 97.3

MEDICATION: Naproxen

ADMISSION DIAGNOSIS
Anemia

PRIMARY COMPLAINT
Tired, feels weak

PATIENT HISTORY

The patient, a 53-year-old white female, was previously diagnosed with non-Hodgkin's lymphoma. She has been coming to the hospital for radiation and chemotherapy treatment. Although she usually feels weak in the days following a treatment session, today she feels especially tired. Previous laboratory results showed a prior steady hemoglobin/hematocrit of 10 g/dL and 30 percent. The patient has had one child and has never been transfused. She is currently taking common prescription medication to reduce back pain and nausea caused by the treatment.

TREATMENT PLAN

Laboratory Tests Ordered: Hemoglobin and hematocrit
Type and cross-match 2 units of red blood cells in case they are needed for transfusion.

PROGRESS REPORTS

11/30/02, 1000: The patient was kept overnight for observation after her chemotherapy.

Treatment Plan: Repeat hemoglobin and hematocrit.

LEARNING ACTIVITIES

PATIENT: Roberta Banks
INSTRUCTIONS: *Before you begin, read the instructions carefully and follow each step in the process.*

STUDY GUIDES

Goal A

The goal in this activity is for you to relate laboratory data with Ms. Banks's symptoms on her admission to the hospital. This learning activity will allow you to collect and assess initial data pertaining to Ms. Banks.

Learning Issues

ISSUE 1: From the clinician's notes, identify relevant signs and symptoms, social and previous medical history, and results of the physical examination.

ISSUE 2: Identify significant laboratory findings that are related to Ms. Banks's clinical condition at the time of presentation. Correlate these findings with her clinical presentation.

ISSUE 3: Review the laboratory test results provided in the documentation and identify discrepancies, if any, that may need to be resolved.

Study Questions A

1. Review the patient's medical records and determine which of the presenting symptoms and which elements of the background history the physician may consider significant in her illness.

CLINICAL SYMPTOMS:

_____

_____

_____

_____

BACKGROUND HISTORY:

_____

_____

_____

_____

2. In the space provided, list the laboratory tests that were requested at the time of Ms. Banks's admission to the facility. Which of the tests requested specifically correlate with her presenting symptoms? Highlight these tests.

_____

_____

_____

_____

3. Now access the laboratory test results from the Laboratory Information System (LIS) in the CD-ROM. Obtain Ms. Banks's laboratory results on admission and record them on the patient laboratory tests results forms provided in this workbook. Review Ms. Banks's laboratory test results at the time of her admission to the hospital.

NOTE: If this is your first time accessing information in the CD-ROM, make sure that you start with "Before you begin."

4. a. Are any of the laboratory test results outside the usual acceptable range? List those results that are outside the usual acceptable range.

b. What do these results indicate?

Goal B

In this portion of the learning activity, the goal is for you to evaluate follow-up measures taken regarding Ms. Banks's condition. This learning activity will allow you to identify discrepancies in laboratory test results and understand how these issues are resolved with additional testing if needed.

Learning Issues

ISSUE 1: Interpret the data obtained and provide the appropriate blood product(s) for this patient.

ISSUE 2: Evaluate the use of the laboratory in this case.

Study Questions B

1. Access the blood bank test results from the LIS in the CD-ROM. Obtain Ms. Banks's laboratory results and record them on the blood bank test results form provided in this workbook. Review the test results and the interpretation of the results provided.

2. a. What is the patient's ABO/Rh group? Do you agree with the ABO/Rh group interpretation?

b. Are there antibodies detected? Are the units cross-matched compatible?

c. What tests should be run in order to investigate the initial test results?

d. What do these test results reveal about the patient?

3. What further studies should be done to resolve the case?

4. What is the transfusion protocol for this patient?

UNIVERSITY MEDICAL CENTER

Name: _____   Date: _____

Record #: _____   Time: _____

ANTIBODY IDENTIFICATION PANEL

Vial	Special Type	Donor	D	C	c	E	e	f	V	Cw	K	k	Kpa	Kpb	Jsa	Jsb	Fya	Fyb	Jka	Jkb	Lea	Leb	P1	M	N	S	s	LUa	LUb	Xga	37	AGH	CC	
						Rh-Hr					Kell						Duffy		Kidd		Lewis		P	MN				Lutheran		Xg	Test Methods			
1	Bg(a+)	R1R1 B1080	+	+	0	0	+	0	0	0	0	+	0	+	0	+	+	0	0	+	0	+	+	+	+	+	+	0	+	+				1
2		R1WR1 B1102	+	+	0	0	+	0	0	+	+	+	0	+	0	+	0	+	+	+	0	+	+	0	+	0	+	0	+	0				2
3	Bg(a+)	R2R2 C1243	+	0	+	+	0	0	0	0	0	+	0	+	0	+	+	+	0	0	0	+	+	+	0	+	+	+	0	+	+				3
4		ROR D575	+	0	+	0	+	+	0	0	0	+	0	+	0	+	0	0	+	+	0	0	+	+	+	0	+	0	+	+				4
5		r'r E370	0	+	+	0	+	+	0	0	0	+	0	+	0	+	+	+	0	+	+	+	+	+	+	+	+	0	+	0				5
6		r'r F416	0	0	+	+	+	+	0	0	0	+	0	+	0	+	+	+	+	+	0	+	0	+	+	0	+	+	+	+				6
7		rrK G488	0	0	+	0	+	+	0	0	+	+	0	+	0	+	0	0	+	+	+	0	0	+	0	0	+	0	+	0				7
8	Yt(b+)	rrFya H347	0	0	+	0	+	+	0	0	0	+	0	+	0	+	+	0	0	0	+	0	+	+	+	+	+	0	+	0				8
9		rr N1434	0	0	+	0	+	+	0	0	0	+	0	+	0	+	+	+	+	+	0	+	+	+	0	+	0	0	+	+				9
10	Co(b+)	R2R2 C199	+	0	+	+	0	0	0	0	0	+	0	+	0	+	+	+	+	0	+	0	+	+	+	0	+	+	+	+				10
TC	He+	R1R2 A1086	+	+	+	+	+	+	0	0	0	+	0	+	0	+	+	+	0	+	0	+	+	+	+	+	+	+	+	0				TC
		Patient's Cells																																

6

UNIVERSITY MEDICAL CENTER

Name: _____   Date: _____

Record #: _____   Time: _____

Cell Tests

Anti-A _____

Anti-B _____

Anti-D IS _____

Anti-D 37 _____

Anti-D AHG _____

Anti-A$_1$ Lectin _____

Serum Tests

A$_1$ Cells _____

A$_2$ Cells _____

B Cells _____

	RT	37	AHG	CC
Screen Cells I	___	___	___	___
Screen Cells II	___	___	___	___
Screen Cells III	___	___	___	___

UNIVERSITY MEDICAL CENTER
CONFIDENTIAL PATIENT INFORMATION
CUMULATIVE SUMMARY REPORT

PATIENT INFORMATION   ID number: _____   Ward: _____

Name: _____   Physician: _____

Address: _____   Date Admitted: _____

_____   Phone: _____

City: _____   State: _____   Zip: _____

Date of Birth: _____   Sex: _____   Race: _____

CHEMISTRY

Tests	Reference Ranges	Date: Time:	Date: Time:	Date: Time:	Date: Time:	Date: Time:
Acid Phos	2.5–11.7 U/L					
ACTH	9–52 pg/mL					
ALT	0–45 IU/L					
Albumin	3.5–5.0 g/dL					
A/G Ratio	0.7–2.1					
Aldosterone	??					
Alkaline Phos	41–137 IU/L					
Ammonia	11–35 μmol/L					
Amylase	95–290 U/L					
Anion Gap	10–18 mmol/L					
AST	0–41 IU/L					
Bilirubin	0.2–1.0 mg/dL					
Bilirubin (direct)	0.2–1.0 mg/dL					
BUN	10–20 mg/dL					
Calcium (total)	4.3–5.3 mEq/L					
Calcuim (ionized)	1.16–1.32 mmol/L					
Chloride	95–100 mmol/L					
Carbon Dioxide	23–32 mmol/L					

CHEMISTRY (page 2)

Tests	Reference Ranges	Date: Time:	Date: Time:	Date: Time:	Date: Time:	Date: Time:
Cholesterol	<200 mg/dL					
CK	15–160 U/L					
CK-MB	15–160 U/L					
Creatinine	0.7–1.5 mg/dL					
Creatintine Clearance	80–120 mL/min					
GGT	6–45 U/L					
Globulin	2.3–3.2 g/dL					
Glucose	65–105 mg/dL					
LD	100–225 U/L					
LDL Cholesterol	75–140 U/L					
LDL/HDL	2.9–2.2					
Lipase	0–1.0 U/mL					
Magnesium	1.3–2.1 mEq/L					
Osmolality	275–295 mOsM/kg					
Phosphorus	2.7–4.5 mg/dL					
Potassium	3.5–5.0 mmol/L					
Protein	5.8–8.2 g/dL					
Sodium	135–145 mmol/L					
Triglycerides	10–190 mg/dL					
Uric Acid	3.5–7.2 mg/dL					
HCO_3	100–225 U/L					

PATIENT INFORMATION   ID number: _____   Ward: _____

Name: _____   Physician: _____

Address: _____   Date Admitted: _____

_____   Phone: _____

City: _____   State: _____   Zip: _____

Date of Birth: _____   Sex: _____   Race: _____

HEMATOLOGY

Test	Reference Ranges	Date: Time:	Date: Time:	Date: Time:	Date: Time:	Date: Time:
Hemoglobin (g/dL)						
Male	14.0–18.0					
Female	12.0–15.0					
Hematocrit (%)						
Male	40–54					
Female	35–49					
RBC ($\times 10^{12}$/L)						
Male	4.6–6.6					
Female	4.0–5.4					
WBC ($\times 10^9$/L)	4.5–11.5					
MCV (fL)	80–94					
MCHC (g/dL or %)	32–36					
MCH (pg)	26–32					
Platelet Count ($\times 10^9$/L)	150–450					
RDW (%)	11.5–14.5					
Reticulocyte Count						
Segmented Neutrophils (%)	50–70					
Lymphocytes (%)	18–42					
Monocytes (%)	2–11					
Basophils (%)	0–2					
Eosinophils (%)	1–3					
Erythrocyte Sed Rate (ESR)						
Male	0–9 mm/hr					
Female	0–15 mm/hr					
Prothrombin Time (PT)	<2-sec deviation from control; 12–14 sec					
Activated Partial Thromboplastin Time (APTT)	<35 sec					
Fibrin Degradation Products (FDP)	4.9 ± 2.8 µg FDP/mL					
Thrombin Time	15 sec					
D-Dimer	<0.5 µg/mL					

CONFIDENTIAL PATIENT INFORMATION
CUMULATIVE SUMMARY REPORT

PATIENT INFORMATION ID number: _____ Ward: _____

Name: _____ Physician: _____

Address: _____ Date Admitted: _____

_____ Phone: _____

City: _____ State: _____ Zip: _____

Date of Birth: _____ Sex: _____ Race: _____

MICROBIOLOGY

Date and Time	Procedure / Specimen	Direct Smear	Preliminary Report	Final Report

CASE SUMMARY

A. Provide a brief summary of possible patient outcomes based on the laboratory test results and the patient's diagnoses.

B. Identify the learning points that you consider helpful in working up this patient's case. *(This will be an individual response.)*

NOTES

PATIENT'S RECORDS

PATIENT NAME: **Joan F. Canaly**

PATIENT IDENTIFICATION NUMBER: **357111**

PHYSICIAN: **Harrison**

PATIENT INFORMATION

NAME: Joan F. Canaly   ID NUMBER: 357111

PHYSICIAN: Harrison

DATE OF OFFICE VISIT: 4/30/00   TIME: 0945

ADDRESS: 2108 Lillie, Ripley, OH 56033

PHONE: 000-193-2003

DATE OF BIRTH: 1/8/65   SEX: F   RACE: W

ADMISSION INFORMATION

WT.: 122 lb   HT.: 5'7"   B/P: 84/68

R: 14   PULSE: 56   TEMP.: 97.5

MEDICATION: Synthroid, 0.05 mg daily

PRIMARY COMPLAINT
Dizziness, "skin getting darker," weight loss, severe fatigue

PATIENT HISTORY
The patient presents stating that she has not felt well for quite some time. She has been increasingly fatigued over the past year. She saw another physician in February 2000 and was found to be hypothyroid; this is being treated successfully with Synthroid. She has had a loss of appetite and a weight loss of 12 lb in the past few months. She complains of light-headedness, especially

with prolonged standing or sitting erect. She finds it difficult to do any of her usual household activities, and she has noticed a distinct darkening of her skin, including the palms of her hands and the soles of her feet. She notes recent mild diarrhea, irregular menstrual periods, and occasional headaches. No fever, chills, or night sweats. No shortness of breath. The patient's past medical history is insignificant except for surgery for a degenerative hip disorder.

FAMILY HISTORY

Father is deceased due to congestive heart failure; mother is cognitively impaired due to head injury.

PHYSICAL EXAMINATION

This patient is thin and frail-appearing for such a young age. No scleral icterus; chest is clear; soft, nontender, nondistended abdomen. Hyperpigmented skin, having the complexion of an African American.

TREATMENT PLAN

Laboratory Tests Ordered: CBC, UA, TP3, ACTH, ALD, COR, CMP
Other Tests Ordered: MRI of head/brain with attention to pituitary, CT scan of adrenals

PROGRESS REPORTS

4/30/00: The patient's hyperpigmentation is strongly suggestive of a disorder of excessive secretion of ACTH. It is uncertain whether this is due to an ACTH-secreting tumor of the CNS or to primary adrenal failure. BP is decreased. Her hypothyroidism is probably related to the current problem as well.

Treatment Plan: ACTH, cortisol, and TSH will be evaluated when results are received. Patient scheduled for recheck and probable referral to endocrinologist.

5/11/00: Referred to endocrinologist as soon as possible.

5/18/00: Endocrinologist's Report:

Review of Symptoms: This is a 35-year-old woman with a greater than 2-year history of generalized fatigue and increased tanning in the past 3 years, with chronic intermittent abdominal pain, dizziness, nausea with rare vomiting, and diarrhea. She complains of a poor sleep pattern, salt cravings, muscle cramping, irritability, hair loss, chronic cold intolerance, and extreme lack of energy. In April her primary-care physician found an elevated potassium, an elevated TSH, and a normal T4.

Physical Examination: A thin white female with severe generalized skin pigmentation and a remarkable face mask. Her blood pressure is 75/50 with a pulse of 104 in the supine position. Her thyroid was small and palpable, with no distinctive nodule.

Treatment Plan: A Cortef/Florinef drug combination will be initiated to replace the decreased mineralocorticoid, and dexamethasone should reduce pigmentation. Synthroid will be continued to treat the primary hypothyroidism.

5/26/00: Patient presents today in follow-up. The patient continues to be very weak and light-headed and fatigues very easily. She continues to be hypotensive, with a BP of 80/60. Patient was advised that it may take some time before an adequate response to her medications is seen. Additional lab tests ordered, as patient is fasting today.

Treatment Plan

Laboratory Tests Ordered: CBC, Chem7, TP3, lipid profile, cardio CRP

6/16/00: Patient is feeling better, with increased weight (134 lb) and blood pressure (110/72). Her energy has improved to some degree. She feels that she should be ready to return to work in a week or two.

Treatment Plan: Continue medications.

7/20/00: Patient returns to office with complaints of edema and swelling of legs, ankles, and hands and shortness of breath that is worse in supine position at night. No cough, sputum production, fever, chills, or chest pain. Electrolytes normal. Fluid overload status and edema are secondary to steroid replacement, and dosage has now been reduced.

Treatment Plan: Lasix ordered for 1 week and then as needed.

Laboratory Tests Ordered: Chem7, CBC, ACTH

11/13/00: Endocrinology Follow-up:

Ms. Canaly seen today for follow-up. Her conditions are well controlled on current medications.

Treatment Plan

Laboratory Tests Ordered: CMP, CBC, ACTH, ALD, COR, UA, TP3
   Schedule visit in 6 months.

LEARNING ACTIVITIES

PATIENT: Joan F. Canaly

INSTRUCTIONS: *Before you begin, read the instructions carefully and follow each step in the process.*

STUDY GUIDES

Goal A

The goal in this activity is for you to relate laboratory data with Ms. Canaly's symptoms, history, diagnosis, and prognosis on the initial office visit. This learning activity will allow you to collect and assess initial data pertaining to Ms. Canaly.

Learning Issues

ISSUE 1: From the clinician's notes, identify relevant signs and symptoms, social and previous medical history, and results of the physical examination.

ISSUE 2: Identify significant laboratory findings that are related to Ms. Canaly's clinical condition at the time of presentation. Correlate these findings with her clinical presentation.

ISSUE 3: Review the laboratory test results provided in the documentation and correlate these data with Ms. Canaly's diagnoses.

Study Questions A

1. Review the patient's medical records and determine which of the presenting symptoms and which elements of the background history the physician may consider significant in her illness.

CLINICAL SYMPTOMS:

BACKGROUND HISTORY:

2. In the space provided, list the laboratory tests that were requested at the time of Ms. Canaly's initial office visit. Which of the tests requested specifically correlate with her presenting symptoms? Highlight these tests.

3. Now access the laboratory test results from the Laboratory Information System (LIS) in the CD-ROM. Obtain Ms. Canaly's initial results and record them on the patient laboratory test results forms provided in this workbook. Review Ms. Canaly's laboratory test results on the date of her initial physician office visit.

    Note: If this is your first time accessing information in the CD-ROM, make sure that you start with "Before you begin."

4. Are any of the laboratory test results outside the usual acceptable range? List those results that are outside the usual acceptable range.

5. a. Which lab results are significant in determining the diagnosis? If so, which ones?

    b. Are any of the lab results at critical levels?

c. What do these results suggest?

_____

_____

_____

_____

d. Do these test results correlate with Ms. Canaly's presenting symptoms? How?

_____

_____

_____

6. Ms. Canaly had been previously diagnosed with primary hypothyroidism and was being treated with Synthroid. Which laboratory test results indicate that her hypothyroidism was not controlled as of 4/30?

_____

_____

_____

_____

Goal B

In this portion of the learning activity, the goal is for you to evaluate follow-up measures taken during the course of Ms. Canaly's illness and how these measures relate to her prognosis and ultimate outcome. This learning activity will allow you to identify reasons for the requests for additional laboratory tests to be performed on this patient.

Learning Issues

ISSUE 1: Interpret the data collected on Ms. Canaly relating to treatment and prognosis.

ISSUE 2: Evaluate the use of the laboratory in this case.

Study Questions B

1. Discuss the regulatory feedback mechanisms between ACTH released from the pituitary gland and cortisol and aldosterone released from the adrenal cortex.

    _____

    _____

    _____

    _____

2. What is the function of aldosterone, and what effect does a decreased concentration of aldosterone produce?

    _____

    _____

    _____

    _____

3. Discuss diurnal variation in ACTH and cortisol concentrations.

    _____

    _____

    _____

    _____

4. a. Does Ms. Canaly have a primary adrenal insufficiency or a secondary pituitary deficiency?

    _____

    _____

    _____

    _____

    b. How can you tell the difference between the two, since they both result in decreased adrenal function?

    _____

    _____

    _____

    _____

    c. Why were a lipid profile and cardio CRP performed on 5/26?

5. Why does Ms. Canaly become light-headed on standing?

6. What is Addisonian crisis?

7. Discuss Schmidt's syndrome.

8. Are there any laboratory tests that have not been ordered on Ms. Canaly that would be helpful in arriving at a more specific diagnosis? If so, what tests do you think were omitted? *(This will be an individual response.)*

9. Discuss the appropriateness of the laboratory tests ordered on Ms. Canaly. Is the laboratory being overutilized or underutilized? Defend your answer. *(This will be an individual response.)*

_____

_____

_____

_____

UNIVERSITY MEDICAL CENTER

Name: _____

Record #: _____

Date: _____

Time: _____

ANTIBODY IDENTIFICATION PANEL

Vial	Special Type	Donor	Rh-Hr								Kell						Duffy		Kidd		Lewis		P	MN				Lutheran		Xg	Test Methods			
			D	C	c	E	e	f	V	Cw	K	k	Kp$_a$	Kp$_b$	Js$_a$	Js$_b$	Fy$_a$	Fy$_b$	Jk$_a$	Jk$_b$	Le$_a$	Le$_b$	P1	M	N	S	s	LU$_a$	LU$_b$	Xg$_a$	37	AGH	CC	
1	Bg(a+)	R1R1 B1080	+	+	0	0	+	0	0	0	0	+	0	+	0	+	+	0	0	+	0	+	+	+	+	+	+	0	+	+				1
2		R1WR1 B1102	+	+	0	0	+	0	0	+	+	+	0	+	0	+	0	+	+	+	0	+	+	0	+	0	+	0	+	0				2
3	Bg(a+)	R2R2 C1243	+	0	+	+	0	0	0	0	0	+	0	+	0	+	+	+	0	+	0	+	+	+	0	+	+	0	+	+				3
4		ROR D575	+	0	+	0	+	+	0	0	0	+	0	+	0	+	0	+	+	0	0	0	+	+	+	0	+	0	+	+				4
5		r'r E370	0	+	+	0	+	+	0	0	0	+	0	+	0	+	+	+	0	+	0	+	+	+	+	+	+	0	+	0				5
6		r"r F416	0	0	+	+	+	+	0	0	0	+	0	+	0	+	+	+	+	+	+	0	+	+	0	0	+	+	+	+				6
7		rrK G488	0	0	+	0	+	+	0	0	+	+	0	+	0	+	0	+	+	0	+	0	0	+	0	0	+	0	+	0				7
8	Yt(b+)	rrFya H347	0	0	+	0	+	+	0	0	0	+	0	+	0	+	+	0	+	+	0	+	+	+	+	+	+	0	+	0				8
9		rr N1434	0	0	+	0	+	+	0	0	0	+	0	+	0	+	+	+	+	+	+	0	0	+	0	0	0	0	+	+				9
10	Co(b+)	R2R2 C199	+	0	+	+	0	0	0	0	0	+	0	+	0	+	+	+	+	0	0	+	0	+	+	+	+	0	+	+				10
TC	He+	R1R2 A1086	+	+	+	+	+	0	0	0	0	+	0	+	0	+	+	+	+	+	0	+	+	+	+	+	+	+	+	0				TC
		Patient's Cells																																

UNIVERSITY MEDICAL CENTER

Name: _____

Date: _____

Record #: _____

Time: _____

Cell Tests

Anti-A _____

Anti-B _____

Anti-D IS _____

Anti-D 37 _____

Anti-D AHG _____

Anti-A$_1$ Lectin _____

Serum Tests

	RT	37	AHG	CC
A$_1$ Cells	_____			
A$_2$ Cells	_____			
B Cells	_____			
Screen Cells I	_____	_____	_____	_____
Screen Cells II	_____	_____	_____	_____
Screen Cells III	_____	_____	_____	_____

UNIVERSITY MEDICAL CENTER
CONFIDENTIAL PATIENT INFORMATION
CUMULATIVE SUMMARY REPORT

PATIENT INFORMATION   ID number: _____   Ward: _____

Name: _____   Physician: _____

Address: _____   Date Admitted: _____

_____   Phone: _____

City: _____   State: _____   Zip: _____

Date of Birth: _____   Sex: _____   Race: _____

CHEMISTRY

Tests	Reference Ranges	Date: Time:	Date: Time:	Date: Time:	Date: Time:	Date: Time:
Acid Phos	2.5–11.7 U/L					
ACTH	9–52 pg/mL					
ALT	0–45 IU/L					
Albumin	3.5–5.0 g/dL					
A/G Ratio	0.7–2.1					
Aldosterone	??					
Alkaline Phos	41–137 IU/L					
Ammonia	11–35 μmol/L					
Amylase	95–290 U/L					
Anion Gap	10–18 mmol/L					
AST	0–41 IU/L					
Bilirubin	0.2–1.0 mg/dL					
Bilirubin (direct)	0.2–1.0 mg/dL					
BUN	10–20 mg/dL					
Calcium (total)	4.3–5.3 mEq/L					
Calcuim (ionized)	1.16–1.32 mmol/L					
Chloride	95–100 mmol/L					
Carbon Dioxide	23–32 mmol/L					

CHEMISTRY (page 2)

Tests	Reference Ranges	Date: Time:	Date: Time:	Date: Time:	Date: Time:	Date: Time:
Cholesterol	<200 mg/dL					
CK	15–160 U/L					
CK-MB	15–160 U/L					
Creatinine	0.7–1.5 mg/dL					
Creatintine Clearance	80–120 mL/min					
GGT	6–45 U/L					
Globulin	2.3–3.2 g/dL					
Glucose	65–105 mg/dL					
LD	100–225 U/L					
LDL Cholesterol	75–140 U/L					
LDL/HDL	2.9–2.2					
Lipase	0–1.0 U/mL					
Magnesium	1.3–2.1 mEq/L					
Osmolality	275–295 mOsM/kg					
Phosphorus	2.7–4.5 mg/dL					
Potassium	3.5–5.0 mmol/L					
Protein	5.8–8.2 g/dL					
Sodium	135–145 mmol/L					
Triglycerides	10–190 mg/dL					
Uric Acid	3.5–7.2 mg/dL					
HCO_3	100–225 U/L					

CONFIDENTIAL PATIENT INFORMATION
CUMULATIVE SUMMARY REPORT

PATIENT INFORMATION   ID number: _____   Ward: _____

Name: _____   Physician: _____

Address: _____   Date Admitted: _____

_____   Phone: _____

City: _____   State: _____   Zip: _____

Date of Birth: _____   Sex: _____   Race: _____

HEMATOLOGY

Test	Reference Ranges	Date: Time:	Date: Time:	Date: Time:	Date: Time:	Date: Time:
Hemoglobin (g/dL) Male Female	14.0–18.0 12.0–15.0					
Hematocrit (%) Male Female	40–54 35–49					
RBC (×10^{12}/L) Male Female	4.6–6.6 4.0–5.4					
WBC (×10^9/L)	4.5–11.5					
MCV (fL)	80–94					
MCHC (g/dL or %)	32–36					
MCH (pg)	26–32					
Platelet Count (×10^9/L)	150–450					
RDW (%)	11.5–14.5					
Reticulocyte Count						
Segmented Neutrophils (%)	50–70					
Lymphocytes (%)	18–42					
Monocytes (%)	2–11					
Basophils (%)	0–2					
Eosinophils (%)	1–3					
Erythrocyte Sed Rate (ESR) Male Female	0–9 mm/hr 0–15 mm/hr					
Prothrombin Time (PT)	<2-sec deviation from control; 12–14 sec					
Activated Partial Thromboplastin Time (APTT)	<35 sec					
Fibrin Degradation Products (FDP)	4.9 ± 2.8 µg FDP/mL					
Thrombin Time	15 sec					
D-Dimer	<0.5 µg/mL					

CONFIDENTIAL PATIENT INFORMATION
CUMULATIVE SUMMARY REPORT

PATIENT INFORMATION   ID number: _____   Ward: _____

Name: _____   Physician: _____

Address: _____   Date Admitted: _____

_____   Phone: _____

City: _____   State: _____   Zip: _____

Date of Birth: _____   Sex: _____   Race: _____

MICROBIOLOGY

Date and Time	Procedure / Specimen	Direct Smear	Preliminary Report	Final Report

CASE SUMMARY

A. Provide a brief summary of possible patient outcomes based on the laboratory test results and the patient's diagnoses.

_____

_____

_____

_____

_____

_____

B. Identify the learning points that you consider helpful in working up this patient's case. *(This will be an individual response.)*

_____

_____

_____

_____

_____

_____

_____

_____

NOTES

_____

_____

_____

_____

_____

_____

▶ PATIENT'S RECORDS

PATIENT NAME: **Michael Carpenter**

PATIENT IDENTIFICATION NUMBER: **369121**

PHYSICIAN: **Holder**

PATIENT INFORMATION

NAME: Michael Carpenter   ID NUMBER: 369121

PHYSICIAN: Holder

DATE OF OFFICE VISIT: 9/26/01   TIME: 1145

ADDRESS: 743 Northern Rd., Lexington, NM 28353

PHONE: 555-555-1000

DATE OF BIRTH: 5/29/66   SEX: M   RACE: W

ADMISSION INFORMATION

WT.: 274 lb   HT.: 5'9"   B/P: 136/110

R: 18   PULSE: 80   TEMP: 97

MEDICATION: Glipizide, 5 mg ×2; Lipitor, 20 mg ×1

ADMISSION DIAGNOSIS

Steatohepatitis

PRIMARY COMPLAINT

Patient was seen in physician's office for routine 6-month checkup, noting increasing fatigue and slight jaundice. Persistent elevations of liver enzymes and bilirubin were noted in previous visits, indicating a possibility of steatohepatitis.

PATIENT HISTORY

Patient has a 2-year history of Type 2 diabetes mellitus and hyperlipidemia. Family has a history of hypertension, increased cholesterol, and heart disease. Patient denies abdominal pain, nausea, vomiting, or drug, alcohol, or tobacco use.

PHYSICAL EXAMINATION

Well-developed, obese white male in no distress; slight jaundice of sclera, regular heart rate and rhythm, clear chest, no abdominal tenderness, liver span approximately 9 cm, no hepatosplenomegaly, slight jaundice in palms of hands.

TREATMENT PLAN

Refer patient to gastroenterology for consult and abdominal ultrasound.
Laboratory Tests Ordered: Hepatic function panel, lipid profile, GGT, ferritin, HgbA1c, CBC

PROGRESS REPORTS

9/26/01, 1530: Patient seen at GI laboratory for abdominal ultrasound and evaluation.

9/28/01: Consultant's Report:

Mildly increased echogenicity throughout the liver, suggesting diffuse fatty infiltration. No focal liver lesions or bile duct dilation. Gallbladder appears normal in size, with no gallstones identified. **Opinion:** Probable fatty infiltration of liver with no other abnormality.

LEARNING ACTIVITIES

PATIENT: **Michael Carpenter**
INSTRUCTIONS: *Before you begin, read the instructions carefully and follow each step in the process.*

STUDY GUIDES

Goal A

The goal in this activity is for you to relate laboratory data with Mr. Carpenter's symptoms, history, diagnosis, and prognosis on this physician visit. This learning activity will allow you to collect and assess initial data pertaining to Mr. Carpenter.

Learning Issues

ISSUE 1: From the clinician's notes, identify relevant signs and symptoms, social and previous medical history, and results of the physical examination.

ISSUE 2: Identify significant laboratory findings that are related to Mr. Carpenter's clinical condition at the time of this physician visit. Correlate these findings with his clinical presentation.

ISSUE 3: Review the laboratory test results provided in the documentation and correlate these data with Mr. Carpenter's diagnoses.

Study Questions A

1. Review the patient's medical records and determine which of the presenting symptoms and which elements of the background history the physician may consider significant in his current illness.

CLINICAL SYMPTOMS:

BACKGROUND HISTORY:

2. In the space provided, list the laboratory tests that were requested at the time of Mr. Carpenter's office visit. Which of the tests requested specifically correlate with his presenting symptoms? Highlight these tests.

3. Now access the laboratory test results from the Laboratory Information System (LIS) in the CD-ROM. Obtain Mr. Carpenter's initial results and record them on the patient laboratory test results forms provided in this workbook. Review Mr. Carpenter's laboratory test results on the day of his current office visit.

   Note: If this is your first time accessing information in the CD-ROM, make sure that you start with "Before you begin."

4. Are any of the laboratory test results at critical levels?

   _____

   _____

   _____

   _____

5. Which laboratory test results indicate a hepatic problem?

   _____

   _____

   _____

6. Do these test results correlate with Mr. Carpenter's presenting symptoms? If so, how do they correlate?

   _____

   _____

   _____

   _____

Goal B

In this portion of the learning activity, the goal is for you to evaluate follow-up measures taken during the course of Mr. Carpenter's illness and how these measures relate to his prognosis and ultimate outcome. This learning activity will allow you to identify reasons for the requests for additional laboratory tests to be performed on this patient.

Learning Issues

ISSUE 1: Interpret the data collected on Mr. Carpenter relating to treatment and prognosis.

ISSUE 2: Evaluate the use of the laboratory in this case.

Study Questions B

1. Mr. Carpenter's abdominal ultrasound indicates fatty infiltration of the liver.

   a. Which of the laboratory tests ordered on 9/26/01 correlate with this diagnosis?

   _____

   _____

   _____

   _____

   b. Interpret the hepatitis panels performed on 9/26/01 and 3/28/00.

   _____

   _____

   _____

   c. Name two additional conditions that could also explain the results on the hepatitis panels.

   _____

   _____

   _____

   d. Why were iron studies performed on 9/26/01?

   _____

   _____

   _____

   _____

2. This patient has a history of Type 2 diabetes mellitus.

   a. Review the laboratory results from previous office visits and list the results that are indicative of this diagnosis.

   _____

   _____

   _____

   _____

   b. What is the significance of Mr. Carpenter's HgbA1c results?

   _____

   _____

   _____

   _____

3. How is Mr. Carpenter being treated for this condition?

   _____

   _____

   _____

4. Is his condition being adequately controlled by the current treatment?

   _____

   _____

   _____

5. How should this patient be followed to ensure that his diabetes is controlled?

   _____

   _____

   _____

   _____

6. What are the long-term complications of uncontrolled diabetes mellitus?

_____

_____

_____

_____

7. This patient also has a history of hyperlipidemia. Review the lipid profile results performed on Mr. Carpenter during the past 2 years. Access the laboratory test results from the LIS in the CD-ROM. Obtain Mr. Carpenter's results and record them on the patient laboratory test results forms provided in this workbook. Review the data.

   a. A significant reduction in Mr. Carpenter's triglyceride concentration is seen between 2/10/00 and 7/14/00. To what do you attribute this?

_____

_____

_____

_____

   b. Are there significant long-term consequences of hyperlipidemia? If so, what are they?

_____

_____

_____

_____

8. Is Mr. Carpenter's risk for coronary artery disease (CAD) increased?

_____

_____

_____

_____

9. Explain the relationship between CAD and decreased serum HDL cholesterol concentrations.

_____

_____

_____

_____

10. The metabolic syndrome is described as a combination of insulin resistance, increased triglycerides, decreased HDL cholesterol, and increased LDL cholesterol concentrations.

   a. Does this diagnosis describe Mr. Carpenter?

   b. What is the likely outcome of a patient with the metabolic syndrome?

   c. Does Mr. Carpenter's lipid concentration contribute to his current complaint of fatty infiltration of the liver?

11. Are there any laboratory tests that have not been ordered on Mr. Carpenter that would be helpful in arriving at a more specific diagnosis? If so, what tests do you think were omitted?

12. Discuss the appropriateness of the laboratory tests ordered on Mr. Carpenter. Is the laboratory being overutilized or underutilized? Defend your answer.

UNIVERSITY MEDICAL CENTER

Name: _____ Date: _____

Record #: _____ Time: _____

ANTIBODY IDENTIFICATION PANEL

Vial	Special Type	Donor	D	C	c	E	e	f	V	Cw	K	k	Kpa	Kpb	Jsa	Jsb	Fya	Fyb	Jka	Jkb	Lea	Leb	P1	M	N	S	s	LUa	LUb	Xga		37	AGH	CC
			|← Rh-Hr →|								|← Kell →|						|Duffy|		|Kidd|		|Lewis|		|P|	|← MN →|				|Lutheran|		|Xg|		|Test Methods|		
1	Bg(a+)	R1R1 B1080	+	+	0	0	+	0	0	0	0	+	0	+	0	+	+	0	0	+	0	+	+	+	+	+	+	0	+	+	1			
2		R1WR1 B1102	+	+	0	0	+	0	0	+	+	+	0	+	0	+	0	+	+	+	0	+	+	0	+	0	+	0	+	0	2			
3	Bg(a+)	R2R2 C1243	+	0	+	+	0	0	0	0	0	+	0	+	0	+	+	+	0	+	0	+	+	+	+	+	+	0	+	+	3			
4		ROR D575	+	0	+	0	+	+	0	0	0	+	0	+	0	+	0	0	+	0	0	0	+	0	+	0	+	0	+	+	4			
5		r'r E370	0	+	+	0	+	+	0	0	0	+	0	+	0	+	+	+	0	+	0	+	+	+	+	+	+	0	+	0	5			
6		r"r F416	0	0	+	+	+	+	0	0	0	+	0	+	0	+	0	+	+	+	0	+	+	+	+	0	+	+	+	+	6			
7		rrK G488	0	0	+	0	+	+	0	0	+	+	0	+	0	+	+	0	0	+	+	0	0	+	0	0	+	0	+	0	7			
8	Yt(b+)	rrFya H347	0	0	+	0	+	+	0	0	0	+	0	+	0	+	+	+	+	0	+	0	+	+	+	+	+	0	+	0	8			
9		rr N1434	0	0	+	0	+	+	0	0	0	+	0	+	0	+	+	+	+	+	0	+	+	+	0	+	0	0	+	+	9			
10	Co(b+)	R2R2 C199	+	0	+	+	0	0	0	0	0	+	0	+	0	+	+	0	+	0	+	0	0	+	+	0	+	0	+	+	10			
TC	He+	R1R2 A1086	+	+	+	+	+	0	0	0	0	+	0	+	0	+	0	0	0	+	0	+	+	+	+	+	+	+	+	0	TC			
		Patient's Cells																																

37

UNIVERSITY MEDICAL CENTER

Name: _____

Record #: _____

Date: _____

Time: _____

Cell Tests

Anti-A _____

Anti-B _____

Anti-D IS _____

Anti-D 37 _____

Anti-D AHG _____

Anti-A_1 Lectin _____

Serum Tests

	RT	37	AHG	CC
A_1 Cells	___			
A_2 Cells	___			
B Cells	___			
Screen Cells I	___	___	___	___
Screen Cells II	___	___	___	___
Screen Cells III	___	___	___	___

UNIVERSITY MEDICAL CENTER
CONFIDENTIAL PATIENT INFORMATION
CUMULATIVE SUMMARY REPORT

PATIENT INFORMATION   ID number: _____   Ward: _____

Name: _____   Physician: _____

Address: _____   Date Admitted: _____

_____   Phone: _____

City: _____   State: _____   Zip: _____

Date of Birth: _____   Sex: _____   Race: _____

CHEMISTRY

Tests	Reference Ranges	Date: Time:	Date: Time:	Date: Time:	Date: Time:	Date: Time:
Acid Phos	2.5–11.7 U/L					
ACTH	9–52 pg/mL					
ALT	0–45 IU/L					
Albumin	3.5–5.0 g/dL					
A/G Ratio	0.7–2.1					
Aldosterone	??					
Alkaline Phos	41–137 IU/L					
Ammonia	11–35 μmol/L					
Amylase	95–290 U/L					
Anion Gap	10–18 mmol/L					
AST	0–41 IU/L					
Bilirubin	0.2–1.0 mg/dL					
Bilirubin (direct)	0.2–1.0 mg/dL					
BUN	10–20 mg/dL					
Calcium (total)	4.3–5.3 mEq/L					
Calcuim (ionized)	1.16–1.32 mmol/L					
Chloride	95–100 mmol/L					
Carbon Dioxide	23–32 mmol/L					

CHEMISTRY (page 2)

Tests	Reference Ranges	Date: Time:	Date: Time:	Date: Time:	Date: Time:	Date: Time:
Cholesterol	<200 mg/dL					
CK	15–160 U/L					
CK-MB	15–160 U/L					
Creatinine	0.7–1.5 mg/dL					
Creatintine Clearance	80–120 mL/min					
GGT	6–45 U/L					
Globulin	2.3–3.2 g/dL					
Glucose	65–105 mg/dL					
LD	100–225 U/L					
LDL Cholesterol	75–140 U/L					
LDL/HDL	2.9–2.2					
Lipase	0–1.0 U/mL					
Magnesium	1.3–2.1 mEq/L					
Osmolality	275–295 mOsM/kg					
Phosphorus	2.7–4.5 mg/dL					
Potassium	3.5–5.0 mmol/L					
Protein	5.8–8.2 g/dL					
Sodium	135–145 mmol/L					
Triglycerides	10–190 mg/dL					
Uric Acid	3.5–7.2 mg/dL					
HCO_3	100–225 U/L					

UNIVERSITY MEDICAL CENTER
CONFIDENTIAL PATIENT INFORMATION
CUMULATIVE SUMMARY REPORT

PATIENT INFORMATION   ID number: _____   Ward: _____

Name: _____   Physician: _____

Address: _____   Date Admitted: _____

_____   Phone: _____

City: _____ State: _____ Zip: _____

Date of Birth: _____ Sex: _____ Race: _____

HEMATOLOGY

Test	Reference Ranges	Date: Time:	Date: Time:	Date: Time:	Date: Time:	Date: Time:
Hemoglobin (g/dL) Male Female	 14.0–18.0 12.0–15.0					
Hematocrit (%) Male Female	 40–54 35–49					
RBC (×10^{12}/L) Male Female	 4.6–6.6 4.0–5.4					
WBC (×10^9/L)	4.5–11.5					
MCV (fL)	80–94					
MCHC (g/dL or %)	32–36					
MCH (pg)	26–32					
Platelet Count (×10^9/L)	150–450					
RDW (%)	11.5–14.5					
Reticulocyte Count						
Segmented Neutrophils (%)	50–70					
Lymphocytes (%)	18–42					
Monocytes (%)	2–11					
Basophils (%)	0–2					
Eosinophils (%)	1–3					
Erythrocyte Sed Rate (ESR) Male Female	 0–9 mm/hr 0–15 mm/hr					
Prothrombin Time (PT)	<2-sec deviation from control; 12–14 sec					
Activated Partial Thromboplastin Time (APTT)	<35 sec					
Fibrin Degradation Products (FDP)	4.9 ± 2.8 µg FDP/mL					
Thrombin Time	15 sec					
D-Dimer	<0.5 µg/mL					

UNIVERSITY MEDICAL CENTER
CONFIDENTIAL PATIENT INFORMATION
CUMULATIVE SUMMARY REPORT

PATIENT INFORMATION   ID number: _____   Ward: _____

Name: _____   Physician: _____

Address: _____   Date Admitted: _____

_____   Phone: _____

City: _____   State: _____   Zip: _____

Date of Birth: _____   Sex: _____   Race: _____

MICROBIOLOGY				
Date and Time	Procedure / Specimen	Direct Smear	Preliminary Report	Final Report

CASE SUMMARY

A. Provide a brief summary of possible patient outcomes based on the laboratory test results and the patient's diagnoses.

_____

_____

_____

_____

_____

_____

_____

B. Identify the learning points you consider helpful in working up this patient's case. *(This will be an individual response.)*

_____

_____

_____

_____

_____

_____

_____

_____

_____

NOTES

_____

_____

_____

_____

_____

_____

_____

▶ PATIENT'S RECORDS

PATIENT NAME: **Deidra Carter**

PATIENT IDENTIFICATION NUMBER: **671450**

PHYSICIAN: **McCarthy**

PATIENT INFORMATION

NAME: Deidra Carter   ID NUMBER: 671450

PHYSICIAN: McCarthy

DATE ADMITTED: 7/30/02   TIME: 0840

ADDRESS: 1230 So. Bench, Ware, VA 22222

PHONE: 000-555-4455

DATE OF BIRTH: 5/5/73   SEX: F   RACE: W

ADMISSION INFORMATION

WT.: 120 lb   HT.: 5'10"   B/P: 130/80

R: 17   PULSE: 90   TEMP.: 97.3

MEDICATION: None

ADMISSION DIAGNOSIS
Broken femur from automobile accident with localized bleeding.

PRIMARY COMPLAINT
Pain in her upper left leg.

PATIENT HISTORY

The patient, a 29-year-old female Caucasian, was taken to the Emergency Department by ambulance after an automobile accident. The patient was the driver of the automobile when the accident occurred. No passengers were in the automobile. The patient hit a patch of ice and skidded off the road into a tree. Paramedics arrived 20 min after the accident. The patient was conscious and alert when first examined by the paramedics. She claimed to have been conscious the entire time following the accident. The patient stated that she felt a sharp pain in her upper left leg. She was worried about her condition, but felt no other physical pain. The paramedics stabilized the damaged leg and transported the patient to the nearest hospital, which was 5 mi away. On arrival at the hospital, the patient was examined. All vital signs appeared normal. A medical history revealed no transfusion history and no pregnancy history. The patient is taking no prescription medications. The patient took two 500-mg aspirin tablets to treat a headache 3 h ago.

TREATMENT PLAN

Laboratory Tests Ordered: Hemoglobin and hematocrit
Other Tests Ordered: X-ray of the damaged leg

PROGRESS REPORTS

7/30/02, 1000: X-ray showed broken left femur.

Treatment Plan: Schedule for surgery. Repair broken left femur and surrounding tissues.

Request 2 units of red blood cells for type and cross-match.

7/30/02, 1800: Patient in recovery. No blood transfusions given.

Treatment Plan:

Laboratory Tests Ordered: Hemoglobin and hematocrit daily for 2 days. If stable, discharge patient. Follow up in orthopedic clinic in 4 weeks.

LEARNING ACTIVITIES

PATIENT: Deidra Carter
INSTRUCTIONS: *Before you begin, read the instructions carefully and follow each step in the process.*

STUDY GUIDES

Goal A

The goal in this activity is for you to relate laboratory data with Ms. Carter's symptoms on her admission to the hospital. This learning activity will allow you to collect and assess initial data pertaining to Ms. Carter.

Learning Issues

Issue 1: From the clinician's notes, identify relevant signs and symptoms, social and previous medical history, and results of the physical examination.

Issue 2: Identify significant laboratory findings that are related to Ms. Carter's clinical condition at the time of presentation. Correlate these findings with her clinical presentation.

Issue 3: Review the laboratory test results provided in the documentation and identify discrepancies, if any, that may need to be resolved.

Study Questions A

1. Review the patient's medical records and determine which of the presenting symptoms and which elements of the background history the physician may consider significant in her illness.

CLINICAL SYMPTOMS:

BACKGROUND HISTORY:

2. In the space provided, list the laboratory tests that were requested at the time of Ms. Carter's admission. Which of the tests requested specifically correlate with her presenting symptoms? Highlight these tests.

_____

_____

_____

_____

3. Now access the laboratory test results from the Laboratory Information System (LIS) in the CD-ROM. Obtain Ms. Carter's laboratory results on admission and record them on the patient laboratory test results forms provided in this workbook. Review Ms. Carter's laboratory test results at the time of her admission to the hospital.

    Note: If this is your first time accessing information in the CD-ROM, make sure that you start with "Before you begin."

4. a. Are any of the laboratory test results outside the usual acceptable ranges? List those results that are outside the usual acceptable ranges.

_____

_____

_____

_____

   b. What do these results indicate?

_____

_____

_____

Goal B

In this portion of the learning activity, the goal is for you to evaluate follow-up measures taken regarding Ms. Carter's condition. This learning activity will allow you to identify discrepancies in laboratory test results and understand how these issues are resolved with additional testing if needed.

Learning Issues

ISSUE 1: Interpret the data obtained and provide the appropriate blood product(s) for this patient.

ISSUE 2: Evaluate the use of the laboratory in this case.

Study Questions B

1. Review the laboratory test results that you obtained from the LIS in Learning Activity A3. Review the ABO/Rh results.

2. How do you interpret the ABO/Rh grouping results?

3. Based on these results, what discrepancies, if any, do you detect? What additional tests can be done to resolve these discrepancies?

4. What information do these test results provide?

5. Are there any other tests to be performed that would confirm the blood type of the patient?

6. How would you determine what red blood cell products to provide for the patient?

7. What red blood cell products should you provide for the patient? Provide a reason for your response.

8. If you tested 100 whole-blood donors,

    a. How many of the donors would be ABO group A?

    b. How many of the ABO group A donors would be ABO subgroup A_2?

    c. How many of the ABO subgroup A_2 donors would produce anti-A_1?

d. How many of the anti-A$_6$ antibodies would be clinically significant?

_____

_____

_____

_____

UNIVERSITY MEDICAL CENTER

Name: _____

Record #: _____

Date: _____

Time: _____

ANTIBODY IDENTIFICATION PANEL

Vial	Special Type	Donor	Rh-Hr								Kell						Duffy		Kidd		Lewis		P	MN				Lutheran		Xg	Test Methods		
			D	C	c	E	e	f	V	Cw	K	k	Kpa	Kpb	Jsa	Jsb	Fya	Fyb	Jka	Jkb	Lea	Leb	P1	M	N	S	s	LUa	LUb	Xga	37	AGH	CC
1	Bg(a+)	R1R1 B1080	+	+	0	0	+	0	0	0	0	+	0	+	0	+	+	0	0	+	0	+	+	+	+	+	+	0	+	+			1
2		R1WR1 B1102	+	+	0	0	+	0	0	+	+	+	0	+	0	+	0	+	+	+	0	+	+	0	+	0	+	0	+	0			2
3	Bg(a+)	R2R2 C1243	+	0	+	+	0	0	0	0	0	+	0	+	0	+	+	+	0	+	0	+	+	+	0	+	+	0	+	+			3
4		ROR D575	+	0	+	0	+	+	0	0	0	+	0	+	0	+	0	0	+	0	0	0	+	+	+	0	+	0	+	+			4
5		r'r E370	0	+	+	0	+	+	0	0	0	+	0	+	0	+	+	+	0	+	0	+	+	+	+	+	+	0	+	0			5
6		r"r F416	0	0	+	+	+	+	0	0	0	+	0	+	0	+	+	+	+	+	0	+	+	+	+	0	+	+	+	+			6
7		rrK G488	0	0	+	0	+	+	0	0	+	+	0	+	0	+	0	+	+	0	+	0	0	+	0	0	+	0	+	0			7
8	Yt(b+)	rrFya H347	0	0	+	0	+	+	0	0	0	+	0	+	0	+	+	0	+	+	+	0	+	+	+	+	+	0	+	+			8
9		rr N1434	0	0	+	0	+	+	0	0	0	+	0	+	0	+	+	+	0	+	0	+	+	+	0	0	0	0	+	+			9
10	Co(b+)	R2R2 C199	+	0	+	+	0	0	0	0	0	+	0	+	0	+	+	+	+	+	+	0	+	+	+	+	+	0	+	+			10
TC	He+	R1R2 A1086	+	+	+	+	+	0	0	0	0	+	0	+	0	+	0	+	0	+	0	+	+	+	+	0	+	+	+	0			TC
		Patient's Cells																															

UNIVERSITY MEDICAL CENTER

Name: _____

Record #: _____

Date: _____

Time: _____

Cell Tests

Anti-A _____

Anti-B _____

Anti-D IS _____

Anti-D 37 _____

Anti-D AHG _____

Anti-A$_1$ Lectin _____

Serum Tests

	RT	37	AHG	CC
A$_1$ Cells	_____			
A$_2$ Cells	_____			
B Cells	_____			
Screen Cells I	_____	_____	_____	_____
Screen Cells II	_____	_____	_____	_____
Screen Cells III	_____	_____	_____	_____

UNIVERSITY MEDICAL CENTER
CONFIDENTIAL PATIENT INFORMATION
CUMULATIVE SUMMARY REPORT

PATIENT INFORMATION   ID number: _____   Ward: _____

Name: _____   Physician: _____

Address: _____   Date Admitted: _____

_____   Phone: _____

City: _____   State: _____   Zip: _____

Date of Birth: _____   Sex: _____   Race: _____

CHEMISTRY

Tests	Reference Ranges	Date: Time:	Date: Time:	Date: Time:	Date: Time:	Date: Time:
Acid Phos	2.5–11.7 U/L					
ACTH	9–52 pg/mL					
ALT	0–45 IU/L					
Albumin	3.5–5.0 g/dL					
A/G Ratio	0.7–2.1					
Aldosterone	??					
Alkaline Phos	41–137 IU/L					
Ammonia	11–35 μmol/L					
Amylase	95–290 U/L					
Anion Gap	10–18 mmol/L					
AST	0–41 IU/L					
Bilirubin	0.2–1.0 mg/dL					
Bilirubin (direct)	0.2–1.0 mg/dL					
BUN	10–20 mg/dL					
Calcium (total)	4.3–5.3 mEq/L					
Calcuim (ionized)	1.16–1.32 mmol/L					
Chloride	95–100 mmol/L					
Carbon Dioxide	23–32 mmol/L					

CHEMISTRY (page 2)

Tests	Reference Ranges	Date: Time:	Date: Time:	Date: Time:	Date: Time:	Date: Time:
Cholesterol	<200					
CK	15–160 U/L					
CK-MB	15–160 U/L					
Creatinine	0.7–1.5 mg/dL					
Creatintine Clearance	80–120 mL/min					
GGT	6–45 U/L					
Globulin	2.3–3.2 g/dL					
Glucose	65–105 mg/dL					
LD	100–225 U/L					
LDL Cholesterol	75–140 U/L					
LDL/HDL	2.9–2.2					
Lipase	0–1.0 U/mL					
Magnesium	1.3–2.1 mEq/L					
Osmolality	275–295mOsM/kg					
Phosphorus	2.7–4.5 mg/dL					
Potassium	3.5–5.0 mmol/L					
Protein	5.8–8.2 g/dL					
Sodium	135–145 mmol/L					
Triglycerides	10–190 mg/dL					
Uric Acid	3.5–7.2 mg/dL					
HCO_3	100–225 U/L					

CONFIDENTIAL PATIENT INFORMATION
CUMULATIVE SUMMARY REPORT

PATIENT INFORMATION   ID number: _____   Ward: _____

Name: _____   Physician: _____

Address: _____   Date Admitted: _____

_____   Phone: _____

City: _____   State: _____   Zip: _____

Date of Birth: _____   Sex: _____   Race: _____

HEMATOLOGY

Test	Reference Ranges	Date: Time:	Date: Time:	Date: Time:	Date: Time:	Date: Time:
Hemoglobin (g/dL) Male Female	14.0–18.0 12.0–15.0					
Hematocrit (%) Male Female	40–54 35–49					
RBC ($\times 10^{12}$/L) Male Female	4.6–6.6 4.0–5.4					
WBC ($\times 10^9$/L)	4.5–11.5					
MCV (fL)	80–94					
MCHC (g/dL or %)	32–36					
MCH (pg)	26–32					
Platelet Count ($\times 10^9$/L)	150–450					
RDW (%)	11.5–14.5					
Reticulocyte Count						
Segmented Neutrophils (%)	50–70					
Lymphocytes (%)	18–42					
Monocytes (%)	2–11					
Basophils (%)	0–2					
Eosinophils (%)	1–3					
Erythrocyte Sed Rate (ESR) Male Female	0–9 mm/hr 0–15 mm/hr					
Prothrombin Time (PT)	<2-sec deviation from control; 12–14 sec					
Activated Partial Thromboplastin Time (APTT)	<35 sec					
Fibrin Degradation Products (FDP)	4.9 ± 2.8 µg FDP/mL					
Thrombin Time	15 sec					
D-Dimer	<0.5 µg/mL					

UNIVERSITY MEDICAL CENTER
CONFIDENTIAL PATIENT INFORMATION
CUMULATIVE SUMMARY REPORT

PATIENT INFORMATION   ID number: _____   Ward: _____

Name: _____   Physician: _____

Address: _____   Date Admitted: _____

_____   Phone: _____

City: _____   State: _____   Zip: _____

Date of Birth: _____   Sex: _____   Race: _____

MICROBIOLOGY

Date and Time	Procedure / Specimen	Direct Smear	Preliminary Report	Final Report

CASE SUMMARY

A. Provide a brief summary of possible patient outcomes based on the laboratory test results and the patient's diagnoses.

B. Identify the learning points that you consider helpful in working up this patient's case *(This will be an individual response.)*

NOTES

▶ PATIENT'S RECORDS

PATIENT NAME: **Robert Chowning**

PATIENT IDENTIFICATION NUMBER: **123435**

PHYSICIAN: **Holly**

PATIENT INFORMATION

NAME: Robert Chowning   ID NUMBER: 123435

PHYSICIAN: Holly

DATE ADMITTED: 1/02/00   TIME: 1300

ADDRESS: 43 Foxtrot St., Isle, TX 78123

PHONE: 210-555-2314

DATE OF BIRTH: 4/18/70   SEX: M   RACE: Hispanic   WARD: 2East

ADMISSION INFORMATION

WT.: 175 lb   HT.: 5'10"   B/P: 110/70

R: 24   PULSE: 120   TEMP: 98.9

MEDICATIONS TAKEN: Amoxicillin

ADMISSION DIAGNOSIS
Pneumonia

PRIMARY COMPLAINT
Cough, diarrhea

PATIENT HISTORY

This patient is a 30-year-old Hispanic male who was brought to the Emergency Department with complaints of cough and greenish sputum production. He reported a sore throat of 2 weeks' duration and fever, nausea, and vomiting for the past 2 days. On the day of admission, he had six episodes of watery diarrhea. The patient also complained of difficulty walking and pain in knee joints, elbows, and wrists. He was treated with amoxicillin 3 days prior to his admission to the hospital.

TREATMENT PLAN

Radiology Ordered: Chest x-ray

Laboratory Tests Ordered: CBC, glucose, BUN, electrolytes, sputum culture and susceptibility

PROGRESS REPORTS

1/02/00, 1800: Mr. Chowning has remained febrile. He continues to experience nausea, vomiting, and diarrhea. His abdomen is soft.

Treatment Plan: Blood cultures × 3 in the a.m. 1 h apart

Stool culture and examination for ova and parasites

1/03/00, 0600: Mr. Chowning continues to cough. He also complains of severe headache and stiff neck, and a petechial rash has appeared on his arms and trunk. There are papular lesions on his face, chest, and lower extremities.

Treatment Plan:

Laboratory Tests Ordered: CBC, PT, PTT, FDP, fibrinogen, platelet count, BUN, electrolytes, creatinine

1/03/00, 0800: Lumbar puncture performed for CSF smear, culture, and susceptibility. CSF studies (CSF glucose, protein, cell count, and differential) to be done.

1/03/00, 1100: The patient shows some unstable mental state; seems confused and hallucinative. His body rash is persistent. The lesions on Mr. Chowning seem to have developed necrosis in some areas, especially in the extremities like fingers and toes. The lesions also appeared gangrenous. Consultation with surgery is required to remove damaged tissues.

Treatment Plan:

Laboratory Tests Ordered: PT, APTT, platelet count

1/04/00, 0600: Meningitis with concurrent bacteremia is confirmed by culture. Blood cultures yield similar organisms. Patient has symptoms of DIC. Started the patient on penicillin IV. Administered FFP, heparin. Electrolyte imbalance is corrected.

Stool cultures and O & P were negative.

Treatment Plan:

Laboratory Tests Ordered: CBC, PT, APTT, electrolytes
Necrotic tissues were surgically removed. PT, APTT normal. Persistent thrombocytopenia is noted.

Follow up with CBC, PT, APTT for 3 days. Repeat blood cultures.

1/10/00: Blood culture results all negative. Discharge patient.

LEARNING ACTIVITIES

PATIENT: **Robert Chowning**
INSTRUCTIONS: *Before you begin, read the instructions carefully and follow each step in the process.*

STUDY GUIDES

Goal A

The goal in this activity is for you to relate laboratory data with Mr. Chowning's symptoms on his admission to the hospital. This learning activity will allow you to collect and assess initial data pertaining to Mr. Chowning.

Learning Issues

ISSUE 1: From the clinician's notes, identify relevant signs and symptoms, social and previous medical history, and results of the physical examination.

ISSUE 2: Identify significant laboratory findings that are related to Mr. Chowning's clinical condition at the time of his admission to the facility. Correlate these findings with his clinical presentation.

Study Questions A

1. Review the patient's medical records and determine which of the presenting symptoms and which elements of the background history the physician may consider significant in his illness.

CLINICAL SYMPTOMS:

_____

_____

_____

_____

BACKGROUND HISTORY:

_____

_____

_____

_____

2. a. In the space provided, list the laboratory tests that were requested at the time of Mr. Chowning's admission to the facility. Which of the tests requested specifically correlate with his presenting symptoms? Highlight these tests.

_____

_____

_____

_____

   b. Why are these tests important in establishing the diagnosis?

_____

_____

_____

_____

3. Now access the laboratory test results from the Laboratory Information System (LIS) in the CD-ROM. Obtain Mr. Chowning's laboratory results on admission and record them on the patient laboratory test results forms provided in this workbook. Review Mr. Chowning's laboratory test results at the time he was admitted to the hospital.
    Note: If this is your first time accessing information in the CD-ROM, make sure that you start with "Before you begin."

4. a. Are any of the CBC results outside the usual acceptable range? List those results that are outside the usual acceptable range. If so, what do these results suggest?

_____

_____

_____

_____

b. Are any of the chemistry results outside the normal acceptable range? If so, what do these test results suggest?

_____

_____

_____

_____

c. How do these test results correlate with Mr. Chowning's presenting symptoms?

_____

_____

_____

_____

5. Go to the Micro Lab in the CD-ROM. Review the microbiology reports.

a. Why was a sputum culture requested? Was a direct sputum smear performed? Why is this important?

_____

_____

_____

_____

b. Review the direct smear interpretation and the work-up of the sputum culture. How do you interpret the microscopic findings of the sputum direct smear? Are the findings significant? Why or why not?

_____

_____

_____

_____

c. What is the result of the sputum culture? Is this an unusual finding? Is this consistent with the direct smear report? What do these results indicate? What clinical implications or decisions may result from this report?

_____

_____

_____

_____

Goal B

In this portion of the learning activity, the goal is for you to evaluate follow-up measures taken during the course of Mr. Chowning's illness and how these measures relate to his prognosis and ultimate outcome. This learning activity will allow you to identify reasons for the requests for additional laboratory tests to be performed on this patient.

Learning Issues

ISSUE 1: Validate the requests for additional laboratory tests.

ISSUE 2: Over the course of Mr. Chowning's illness, analyze the events that led to his current condition.

Study Questions B

1. Review Mr. Chowning's progress reports.

   a. List the additional tests requested by the physician.

   _____

   _____

   _____

   b. On what in Mr. Chowning's clinical progress (i.e., his signs and symptoms) did the clinician base the request for coagulation studies, blood cultures, and stool examinations?

   _____

   _____

   _____

   c. On what in Mr. Chowning's clinical condition did the clinician base the request for CSF studies, direct smear, and culture?

   _____

   _____

   _____

2. Go back to the CD-ROM. Obtain the results of the coagulation studies, CSF hematology, and chemistry tests. Record the test results on the patient laboratory test results forms provided in this workbook. Review Mr. Chowning's CSF hematology and chemistry tests.

3. a. What do the results of the coagulation studies indicate? Explain the implications of your findings.

_____

_____

_____

_____

    b. What do the CSF hematology and chemistry test findings indicate? Do they support the clinical diagnosis?

_____

_____

_____

_____

4. Go to the micro lab in the CD-ROM and review the CSF direct smear results and CSF culture work-up. Review the blood and stool culture results and other findings. Record the results and the interpretations of these results.

_____

_____

_____

_____

    a. How do you interpret the CSF direct smear? Are your findings significant? Why or why not?

_____

_____

_____

_____

    b. What is the result of the CSF culture? Is this consistent with the direct smear results? How do the blood culture results correlate with the other laboratory findings and the patient's clinical presentation?

_____

_____

_____

_____

c. Why is meningococcemia considered to be one of the most serious systemic infections?

_____

_____

_____

_____

d. What are possible outcomes for this patient, based on your findings?

_____

_____

_____

_____

Name: _____

Date: _____

Record #: _____

Time: _____

ANTIBODY IDENTIFICATION PANEL

Vial	Special Type	Donor	D	C	c	E	e	f	V	Cw	K	k	Kp_a	Kp_b	Js_a	Js_b	Fy_a	Fy_b	Jk_a	Jk_b	Le_a	Le_b	P1	M	N	S	s	LU_a	LU_b	Xg_a	37	AGH	CC
1	Bg(a+)	R1R1 B1080	+	+	0	0	+	0	0	0	0	+	0	+	0	+	+	0	0	+	0	+	+	+	+	+	+	0	+	+				1
2		R1WR1 B1102	+	+	0	0	+	0	0	+	+	+	0	+	0	+	0	+	+	+	0	+	+	0	+	0	+	0	+	0				2
3	Bg(a+)	R2R2 C1243	+	0	+	+	0	0	0	0	0	+	0	+	0	+	+	+	0	+	0	0	+	+	0	+	+	0	+	+				3
4		ROR D575	+	0	+	0	+	+	0	0	0	+	0	+	0	+	0	0	+	0	0	0	+	+	+	0	+	0	+	+				4
5		r'r E370	0	+	+	0	+	+	0	0	0	+	0	+	0	+	+	+	0	+	0	+	+	+	+	+	+	0	+	0				5
6		r"r F416	0	0	+	+	+	+	0	0	0	+	0	+	0	+	0	+	+	+	0	0	0	+	+	0	+	+	+	+				6
7		rrK G488	0	0	+	0	+	+	0	0	+	+	0	+	0	+	0	0	0	+	+	0	+	0	+	0	+	0	+	0				7
8	Yt(b+)	rrFya H347	0	0	+	0	+	+	0	0	0	+	0	+	0	+	+	0	+	0	+	0	+	+	+	+	+	0	+	0				8
9		rr N1434	0	0	+	0	+	+	0	0	0	+	0	+	0	+	+	+	+	+	0	+	0	+	0	+	0	0	+	+				9
10	Co(b+)	R2R2 C199	+	0	+	+	0	0	0	0	0	+	0	+	0	+	+	+	0	0	+	0	+	+	+	0	+	0	+	+				10
TC	He+	R1R2 A1086	+	+	+	+	+	0	0	0	0	+	0	+	0	+	0	0	+	+	0	+	+	+	+	+	+	+	+	0				TC
		Patient's Cells																															

67

UNIVERSITY MEDICAL CENTER

Name: _____

Record #: _____

Date: _____

Time: _____

Cell Tests

Anti-A _____

Anti-B _____

Anti-D IS _____

Anti-D 37 _____

Anti-D AHG _____

Anti-A_1 Lectin _____

Serum Tests

	RT	37	AHG	CC
A_1 Cells	_____			
A_2 Cells	_____			
B Cells	_____			
Screen Cells I	_____	_____	_____	_____
Screen Cells II	_____	_____	_____	_____
Screen Cells III	_____	_____	_____	_____

UNIVERSITY MEDICAL CENTER
CONFIDENTIAL PATIENT INFORMATION
CUMULATIVE SUMMARY REPORT

PATIENT INFORMATION ID number: _____ Ward: _____

Name: _____ Physician: _____

Address: _____ Date Admitted: _____

_____ Phone: _____

City: _____ State: _____ Zip: _____

Date of Birth: _____ Sex: _____ Race: _____

CHEMISTRY

Tests	Reference Ranges	Date: Time:	Date: Time:	Date: Time:	Date: Time:	Date: Time:
Acid Phos	2.5–11.7 U/L					
ACTH	9–52 pg/mL					
ALT	0–45 IU/L					
Albumin	3.5–5.0 g/dL					
A/G Ratio	0.7–2.1					
Aldosterone	??					
Alkaline Phos	41–137 IU/L					
Ammonia	11–35 µmol/L					
Amylase	95–290 U/L					
Anion Gap	10–18 mmol/L					
AST	0–41 IU/L					
Bilirubin	0.2–1.0 mg/dL					
Bilirubin (direct)	0.2–1.0 mg/dL					
BUN	10–20 mg/dL					
Calcium (total)	4.3–5.3 mEq/L					
Calcuim (ionized)	1.16–1.32 mmol/L					
Chloride	95–100 mmol/L					
Carbon Dioxide	23–32 mmol/L					

CHEMISTRY (page 2)

Tests	Reference Ranges	Date: Time:	Date: Time:	Date: Time:	Date: Time:	Date: Time:
Cholesterol	<200 mg/dL					
CK	15–160 U/L					
CK-MB	15–160 U/L					
Creatinine	0.7–1.5 mg/dL					
Creatintine Clearance	80–120 mL/min					
GGT	6–45 U/L					
Globulin	2.3–3.2 g/dL					
Glucose	65–105 mg/dL					
LD	100–225 U/L					
LDL Cholesterol	75–140 U/L					
LDL/HDL	2.9–2.2					
Lipase	0–1.0 U/mL					
Magnesium	1.3–2.1 mEq/L					
Osmolality	275–295 mOsM/kg					
Phosphorus	2.7–4.5 mg/dL					
Potassium	3.5–5.0 mmol/L					
Protein	5.8–8.2 g/dL					
Sodium	135–145 mmol/L					
Triglycerides	10–190 mg/dL					
Uric Acid	3.5–7.2 mg/dL					
HCO_3	100–225 U/L					

PATIENT INFORMATION ID number: _____ Ward: _____

Name: _____ Physician: _____

Address: _____ Date Admitted: _____

_____ Phone: _____

City: _____ State: _____ Zip: _____

Date of Birth: _____ Sex: _____ Race: _____

HEMATOLOGY

Test	Reference Ranges	Date: Time:	Date: Time:	Date: Time:	Date: Time:	Date: Time:
Hemoglobin (g/dL) Male Female	14.0–18.0 12.0–15.0					
Hematocrit (%) Male Female	40–54 35–49					
RBC ($\times 10^{12}$/L) Male Female	4.6–6.6 4.0–5.4					
WBC ($\times 10^{9}$/L)	4.5–11.5					
MCV (fL)	80–94					
MCHC (g/dL or %)	32–36					
MCH (pg)	26–32					
Platelet Count ($\times 10^{9}$/L)	150–450					
RDW (%)	11.5–14.5					
Reticulocyte Count						
Segmented Neutrophils (%)	50–70					
Lymphocytes (%)	18–42					
Monocytes (%)	2–11					
Basophils (%)	0–2					
Eosinophils (%)	1–3					
Erythrocyte Sed Rate (ESR) Male Female	0–9 mm/hr 0–15 mm/hr					
Prothrombin Time (PT)	<2-sec deviation from control; 12–14 sec					
Activated Partial Thromboplastin Time (APTT)	<35 sec					
Fibrin Degradation Products (FDP)	4.9 ± 2.8 µg FDP/mL					
Thrombin Time	15 sec					
D-Dimer	<0.5 µg/mL					

UNIVERSITY MEDICAL CENTER
CONFIDENTIAL PATIENT INFORMATION
CUMULATIVE SUMMARY REPORT

PATIENT INFORMATION   ID number: _____   Ward: _____

Name: _____   Physician: _____

Address: _____   Date Admitted: _____

_____   Phone: _____

City: _____   State: _____   Zip: _____

Date of Birth: _____   Sex: _____   Race: _____

MICROBIOLOGY

Date and Time	Procedure / Specimen	Direct Smear	Preliminary Report	Final Report

CASE SUMMARY

A. Provide a brief summary of possible patient outcomes based on the laboratory test results and the patient's diagnoses.

B. Identify the learning points that you consider helpful in working up this patient's case. *(This will be an individual response.)*

NOTES

► PATIENT'S RECORDS

PATIENT NAME: **Angelina Cortez**

PATIENT IDENTIFICATION NUMBER: **123487**

PHYSICIAN: **Cosby**

PATIENT INFORMATION

NAME: Angelina Cortez   ID NUMBER: 123487

PHYSICIAN: Cosby

ADMISSION: 02/09/01   TIME: 1300

ADDRESS: 2650 Dunno St., Noware, ND 80983

PHONE: 211-111-2222

DATE OF BIRTH: 7/13/88   SEX: F   RACE: Hispanic   WARD: 4W

ADMISSION INFORMATION

WT.: 100 lb   HT.: 4'6"   B/P: 102/71

R: 24   PULSE: 122   TEMP.: 101.2

ADMISSION DIAGNOSIS

Thrombocytopenia

PRIMARY COMPLAINT

Fever, fatigue, anorexia, unexplained bruises

PATIENT HISTORY

The patient is a 13-year-old female who was seen at the clinic because of complaints of fever, fatigue, and decreased appetite for the past 2½ weeks. She also complained of easy bruising, especially on arms and legs. On physical

75

examination, the patient showed pallor, was febrile, and appeared weak and lethargic. The patient also revealed petechiae over her mouth, ecchymoses, and signs of weight loss, which had occurred over the last 6 months.

TREATMENT PLAN

Laboratory Tests Ordered: CBC, electrolytes, glucose, BUN

PROGRESS REPORTS

02/12/01, 1800: The patient was given 6 units of platelets and 250 mL of packed RBC followed by 10 mg of Lasix IV. The patient became stabilized.

Treatment Plan: Evaluate lab results. Request bone marrow aspiration and immunologic markers.

02/22/01, 0600: The patient was placed on chemotherapy.

Treatment Plan: Hemoglobin, hematocrit, platelet count daily. Transfuse platelets and packed red blood cells as needed.

03/19/01, 0900:

Treatment Plan: Discharge patient. Follow up in outpatient clinic.

LEARNING ACTIVITIES

PATIENT: Angelina Cortez

INSTRUCTIONS: *Before you begin, read the instructions carefully and follow each step in the process.*

STUDY GUIDES

Goal A

The goal in this activity is for you to relate laboratory data with Ms. Cortez's symptoms on her admission to the hospital. This learning activity will allow you to collect and assess initial data pertaining to Ms. Cortez.

Learning Issues

ISSUE 1: Identify clinical symptoms that indicate Ms. Cortez's condition based on her history.

ISSUE 2: Determine why immunologic marker results are significant parameters in monitoring this disease process.

ISSUE 3: Consider the significance of the request for CSF and bone marrow studies.

Study Questions A

1. Review the patient's medical records and determine which of the presenting symptoms and which elements of the background history the physician may consider significant in her illness.

CLINICAL SYMPTOMS:

_____

_____

_____

_____

BACKGROUND HISTORY:

_____

_____

_____

_____

2. In the space provided, list the laboratory tests requested at the time of Ms. Cortez's admission to the facility. Which of the tests requested specifically correlate with her presenting symptoms? Highlight these tests.

_____

_____

_____

_____

3. Now access the laboratory test results from the Laboratory Information System (LIS) in the CD-ROM. Obtain Ms. Cortez's laboratory result on admission and record them on the patient laboratory tests results forms provided in this workbook. Review Ms. Cortez's laboratory test results at the time she was admitted to the hospital.

   Note: If this is your first time accessing information in the CD-ROM, make sure that you start with "Before you begin."

4. a. Are any of the laboratory test results outside the usual acceptable range? If so, what do these results suggest?

    b. How do these test results correlate with Ms. Cortez's presenting symptoms?

5. Are there other laboratory findings that you consider significant in this case, given the background history of the patient?

Goal B

In this portion of the learning activity, the goal is for you to evaluate the patient's laboratory test results and determine how these results relate to her prognosis and ultimate outcome.

Learning Issues

ISSUE 1: Consider the consequences that may result if Ms. Cortez's condition remains undetected.

ISSUE 2: Evaluate the use of the laboratory in this case.

Study Questions B

1. a. Which of the laboratory test results support, confirm, or reject the initial diagnosis?

   b. Review the peripheral blood smear results. Use the **CD-ROM** to access the hematology findings. What morphologic characteristics led to the diagnosis of this patient's condition?

   c. How is the investigation carried out to confirm the diagnosis?

2. How do cell surface markers differentiate this disease condition from others?

3. Why are chromosomal analyses important as diagnostic and prognostic markers?

4. What is the prognosis for this patient, given her age and diagnosis?

Name: _____ Date: _____

Record #: _____ Time: _____

ANTIBODY IDENTIFICATION PANEL

Vial	Special Type	Donor	Rh-Hr								Kell						Duffy		Kidd		Lewis		P	MN				Lutheran		Xg		Test Methods		
			D	C	c	E	e	f	V	Cw	K	k	Kp$_a$	Kp$_b$	Js$_a$	Js$_b$	Fy$_a$	Fy$_b$	Jk$_a$	Jk$_b$	Le$_a$	Le$_b$	P1	M	N	S	s	LU$_a$	LU$_b$	Xg$_a$	37	AGH	CC
1	Bg(a+)	R1R1 B1080	+	+	0	0	+	0	0	0	0	+	0	+	0	+	+	0	0	+	0	+	+	+	+	+	+	0	+	+	1			
2		R1WR1 B1102	+	+	0	0	+	0	0	+	+	+	0	+	0	+	0	+	+	+	0	+	+	0	+	0	+	0	+	0	2			
3	Bg(a+)	R2R2 C1243	+	0	+	+	0	0	0	0	0	+	0	+	0	+	+	+	+	+	0	0	+	+	0	+	+	0	+	+	3			
4		ROR D575	+	0	+	0	+	+	0	0	0	+	0	+	0	+	0	0	0	0	0	0	+	+	+	0	+	0	+	+	4			
5		r'r E370	0	+	+	0	+	+	0	0	0	+	0	+	0	+	0	+	+	+	0	+	+	+	+	+	+	0	+	0	5			
6		r"r F416	0	0	+	+	+	+	0	0	0	+	0	+	0	+	0	+	+	+	+	0	0	+	+	0	+	0	+	+	6			
7		rrK G488	0	0	+	0	+	+	0	0	+	+	0	+	0	+	+	+	0	0	+	0	0	+	0	0	+	0	+	0	7			
8	Yt(b+)	rrFya H347	0	0	+	0	+	+	0	0	0	+	0	+	0	+	+	0	+	+	+	0	+	+	+	+	+	0	+	0	8			
9		rr N1434	0	0	+	0	+	+	0	0	0	+	0	+	0	+	+	+	+	0	0	0	+	+	0	+	0	0	+	+	9			
10	Co(b+)	R2R2 C199	+	0	+	+	0	0	0	0	0	+	0	+	0	+	+	+	0	0	0	0	0	+	+	0	+	0	+	+	10			
TC	He+	R1R2 A1086	+	+	+	+	+	0	0	0	0	+	0	+	0	+	0	0	0	+	0	+	+	+	+	+	+	+	+	0	TC			
		Patient's Cells																																	

UNIVERSITY MEDICAL CENTER

Name: _____

Record #: _____

Date: _____

Time: _____

Cell Tests

Anti-A _____

Anti-B _____

Anti-D IS _____

Anti-D 37 _____

Anti-D AHG _____

Anti-A_1 Lectin _____

Serum Tests

A_1 Cells _____

A_2 Cells _____

B Cells _____

	RT	37	AHG	CC
Screen Cells I	___	___	___	___
Screen Cells II	___	___	___	___
Screen Cells III	___	___	___	___

ANGELINA CORTEZ

UNIVERSITY MEDICAL CENTER
CONFIDENTIAL PATIENT INFORMATION
CUMULATIVE SUMMARY REPORT

PATIENT INFORMATION   ID number: _____   Ward: _____

Name: _____   Physician: _____

Address: _____   Date Admitted: _____

_____   Phone: _____

City: _____ State: _____ Zip: _____

Date of Birth: _____ Sex: _____ Race: _____

CHEMISTRY

Tests	Reference Ranges	Date: Time:	Date: Time:	Date: Time:	Date: Time:	Date: Time:
Acid Phos	2.5–11.7 U/L					
ACTH	9–52 pg/mL					
ALT	0–45 IU/L					
Albumin	3.5–5.0 g/dL					
A/G Ratio	0.7–2.1					
Aldosterone	??					
Alkaline Phos	41–137 IU/L					
Ammonia	11–35 μmol/L					
Amylase	95–290 U/L					
Anion Gap	10–18 mmol/L					
AST	0–41 IU/L					
Bilirubin	0.2–1.0 mg/dL					
Bilirubin (direct)	0.2–1.0 mg/dL					
BUN	10–20 mg/dL					
Calcium (total)	4.3–5.3 mEq/L					
Calcuim (ionized)	1.16–1.32 mmol/L					
Chloride	95–100 mmol/L					
Carbon Dioxide	23–32 mmol/L					

CHEMISTRY (page 2)

Tests	Reference Ranges	Date: Time:	Date: Time:	Date: Time:	Date: Time:	Date: Time:
Cholesterol	<200 mg/dL					
CK	15–160 U/L					
CK-MB	15–160 U/L					
Creatinine	0.7–1.5 mg/dL					
Creatintine Clearance	80–120 mL/min					
GGT	6–45 U/L					
Globulin	2.3–3.2 g/dL					
Glucose	65–105 mg/dL					
LD	100–225 U/L					
LDL Cholesterol	75–140 U/L					
LDL/HDL	2.9–2.2					
Lipase	0–1.0 U/mL					
Magnesium	1.3–2.1 mEq/L					
Osmolality	275–295 mOsM/kg					
Phosphorus	2.7–4.5 mg/dL					
Potassium	3.5–5.0 mmol/L					
Protein	5.8–8.2 g/dL					
Sodium	135–145 mmol/L					
Triglycerides	10–190 mg/dL					
Uric Acid	3.5–7.2 mg/dL					
HCO_3	100–225 U/L					

CONFIDENTIAL PATIENT INFORMATION
CUMULATIVE SUMMARY REPORT

PATIENT INFORMATION

ID number: _____   Ward: _____

Name: _____   Physician: _____

Address: _____   Date Admitted: _____

_____   Phone: _____

City: _____   State: _____   Zip: _____

Date of Birth: _____   Sex: _____   Race: _____

HEMATOLOGY

Test	Reference Ranges	Date: Time:	Date: Time:	Date: Time:	Date: Time:	Date: Time:
Hemoglobin (g/dL) Male Female	 14.0–18.0 12.0–15.0					
Hematocrit (%) Male Female	 40–54 35–49					
RBC ($\times 10^{12}$/L) Male Female	 4.6–6.6 4.0–5.4					
WBC ($\times 10^{9}$/L)	4.5–11.5					
MCV (fL)	80–94					
MCHC (g/dL or %)	32–36					
MCH (pg)	26–32					
Platelet Count ($\times 10^{9}$/L)	150–450					
RDW (%)	11.5–14.5					
Reticulocyte Count						
Segmented Neutrophils (%)	50–70					
Lymphocytes (%)	18–42					
Monocytes (%)	2–11					
Basophils (%)	0–2					
Eosinophils (%)	1–3					
Erythrocyte Sed Rate (ESR) Male Female	 0–9 mm/hr 0–15 mm/hr					
Prothrombin Time (PT)	<2-sec deviation from control; 12–14 sec					
Activated Partial Thromboplastin Time (APTT)	<35 sec					
Fibrin Degradation Products (FDP)	4.9 ± 2.8 µg FDP/mL					
Thrombin Time	15 sec					
D-Dimer	<0.5 µg/mL					

UNIVERSITY MEDICAL CENTER
CONFIDENTIAL PATIENT INFORMATION
CUMULATIVE SUMMARY REPORT

PATIENT INFORMATION   ID number: _____   Ward: _____

Name: _____   Physician: _____

Address: _____   Date Admitted: _____

_____   Phone: _____

City: _____   State: _____   Zip: _____

Date of Birth: _____   Sex: _____   Race: _____

MICROBIOLOGY

Date and Time	Procedure / Specimen	Direct Smear	Preliminary Report	Final Report

CASE SUMMARY

A. Provide a brief summary of possible patient outcomes based on the laboratory test results and the patient's diagnoses.

B. Identify the learning points that you consider helpful in working up this patient's case. *(This will be an individual response.)*

NOTES

► PATIENT'S RECORDS

PATIENT NAME: **Michelle Craig**

PATIENT IDENTIFICATION NUMBER: **370116**

PHYSICIAN: **Stark**

DIAGNOSIS 1

PATIENT INFORMATION

NAME: Michelle Craig   ID NUMBER: 370116

PHYSICIAN: Stark

DATE ADMITTED: 1/28/94

ADDRESS: 354 Hodges, Chicago, IL 02425

PHONE: 000-555-3892

DATE OF BIRTH: 12/13/69   SEX: F   RACE: W

ADMISSION INFORMATION

WT.: 121 lb   HT.: 5'6"   B/P: 126/70

R: 16   PULSE: 88   TEMP.: 98.0

MEDICATION: None

ADMISSION DIAGNOSIS

Gastroenteritis with dehydration

PRIMARY COMPLAINT

Ten-day history of nausea with vomiting, diarrhea, cough, and congestion

PATIENT HISTORY

Ms. Craig is a 24-year-old white female with a 10-day history of viral syndrome. Her symptoms progressively worsened, and she presented to the ED. She was noted to have some petechial lesions of the lower extremities and appeared to be significantly dehydrated, and was admitted for further evaluation and treatment.

PROGRESS REPORTS

1/28/94:   Ms. Craig was admitted for treatment of gastroenteritis with dehydration as well as thrombocytopenia. Her initial treatment included administration of IV fluids, antiemetics, and ciprofloxacin. She was transfused with 10 units of platelets, but this increased her platelet count only from 12,000/μL to 14,000/μL.

Treatment Plan:

Laboratory Tests Ordered: CBC, CMP, urinalysis, platelet count

1/29/94: A hematology consult was obtained. She was placed on IV Solu-Medrol. The follow-up platelet count was 10,000/μL, and she was given another 10 units of platelets.

Treatment Plan:

Laboratory Tests Ordered: Platelet count, iron profile, retic, sedimentation rate, hepatitis profile, urine culture

1/30/94: The patient's pulmonary congestion continued, and a chest x-ray revealed an atypical pneumonia. She became hypoxic and was transferred to the transitional care unit for close hemodynamic monitoring. She was placed on supplemental oxygen and additional antibiotics. Though Ms. Craig had no symptoms consistent with lupus, the results of positive FANA, CRP, and sedimentation rate warranted further consideration of this diagnosis.

Treatment Plan:

Laboratory Tests Ordered: Platelet count, rheumatology profile, CMP
Other Tests Ordered: Chest x-ray, echocardiogram, CT of abdomen

1/31/94: Twenty units of platelets were transfused.

Treatment Plan:

Laboratory Tests Ordered: Platelet count

2/1/94: A rheumatology consult was obtained, and as a result Ms. Craig received pulse doses of steroids. Ten units of platelets were transfused.

Treatment Plan:

Laboratory Tests Ordered: CBC, antinuclear antibody profile

2/2/94: Consulting Physician's Report:

Positive antinuclear antibody test with a titer of greater than 1:320 with a speckled and rim pattern. Positive anti-double-stranded DNA. Mild decrease in complement and increased titers to anti-Sm and anti-RNP.

Ms. Craig demonstrated an excellent clinical response to the steroid treatment, and her platelet count rose to 62,000/μL.

Treatment Plan:

Laboratory Tests Ordered: Platelet count

2/4/94: Ms. Craig was transferred to the regular floor on February 4, and she converted to oral prednisone.

Treatment Plan:

Laboratory Tests Ordered: Platelet count, CMP, sedimentation rate
Other Tests Ordered: Chest x-ray

2/6/94: Ms. Craig's activity level and appetite were increased on February 6, and her platelet counts and CBC were stable. Ms. Craig was discharged with instructions to follow a regular diet, resume activities as tolerated, and follow up with her primary-care physician in 1 week.

Treatment Plan:

Laboratory Tests Ordered: CBC
Discharge Medications:
   1. Prednisone
   2. Biaxin
Discharge Diagnosis:
   1. Thrombocytopenia
   2. Systemic lupus erythematosis
   3. Gastroenteritis with dehydration
   4. Lupus vasculitis

LEARNING ACTIVITIES

PATIENT: **Michelle Craig**
INSTRUCTIONS: *Before you begin, read the instructions carefully and follow each step in the process.*

STUDY GUIDES

Goal A

The goal in this activity is for you to relate laboratory data with Ms. Craig's symptoms, history, diagnosis, and prognosis on her admission to the hospital. This learning activity will allow you to collect and assess initial data pertaining to Ms. Craig.

Learning Issues

ISSUE 1: From the clinician's notes, identify relevant signs and symptoms, social and previous medical history, and results of the physical examination.

ISSUE 2: Identify significant laboratory findings that are related to Ms. Craig's clinical condition at the time of presentation. Correlate these findings with her clinical presentation.

ISSUE 3: Review the laboratory test results provided in the documentation and correlate these data with Ms. Craig's diagnoses.

Study Questions A

1. Review the patient's medical records and determine which of the presenting symptoms and which elements of the background history the physician may consider significant in her illness.

CLINICAL SYMPTOMS:

_____

_____

_____

_____

BACKGROUND HISTORY:

_____

_____

_____

_____

2. In the space provided, list the laboratory tests that were requested at the time of Ms. Craig's admission. Which of the tests requested specifically correlate with her presenting symptoms? Highlight these tests.

_____

_____

_____

_____

3. Now access the laboratory test results from the Laboratory Information System (LIS) in the CD-ROM. Obtain Ms. Craig's results and record them on the patient laboratory test results forms provided in this workbook. Review Ms. Craig's laboratory test results at admission.

    Note: If this is your first time accessing information in the CD-ROM, make sure that you start with "Before you begin."

4. Are any of the laboratory test results outside the usual acceptable range? List those results that are outside the usual acceptable range.

    _____

    _____

    _____

    _____

5. a. Are any of the lab results at critical levels?

    _____

    _____

    _____

    b. What do these results suggest?

    _____

    _____

    _____

    c. Do these test results correlate with Ms. Craig's presenting symptoms? How?

    _____

    _____

    _____

Goal B

In this portion of the learning activity, the goal is for you to evaluate follow-up measures taken during the course of Ms. Craig's illness and how these measures relate to her prognosis and ultimate outcome. This learning activity will allow you to identify reasons for the requests for additional laboratory tests to be performed on this patient.

Learning Issues

ISSUE 1: Interpret the data collected on Ms. Craig relating to treatment and prognosis.

ISSUE 2: Evaluate the use of the laboratory in this case.

Study Questions B

1. What are the most common causes of anemia?

2. What are the most common causes of thrombocytopenia?

3. Is Ms. Craig suspected of any of the conditions described in Questions 1 and 2?

4. Describe the symptoms of SLE.

5. What led Ms. Craig's physicians to investigate the possibility of SLE?

6. Why did Ms. Craig's platelet count remain unchanged after her numerous platelet transfusions?

7. Why did Ms. Craig's thrombocytopenia respond to steroid therapy?

8. What are the complications for a patient with long-term SLE?

9. How should Ms. Craig be followed for progression of her disease?

10. a. Do any of Ms. Craig's laboratory tests indicate kidney damage?

    b. How do you explain the increased BUN on admission?

11. Explain the results of the C-reactive protein performed on Ms. Craig on 1/29.

12. Explain the results of the ANA profile performed on Ms. Craig on 2/1.

13. a. Why was an iron profile ordered?

b. What is Ms. Craig's result on the iron profile?

c. What do these results indicate?

14. Are there any laboratory tests that have not been ordered on Ms. Craig that would be helpful in arriving at a more specific diagnosis? If so, what tests do you think were omitted?

15. Discuss the appropriateness of the laboratory tests ordered on Ms. Craig. Is the laboratory being overutilized or underutilized? Defend your answer.

UNIVERSITY MEDICAL CENTER

Name: _____

Record #: _____

Date: _____

Time: _____

ANTIBODY IDENTIFICATION PANEL

Vial	Special Type	Donor	Rh-Hr								Kell						Duffy		Kidd		Lewis		P	MN				Lutheran		Xg	Test Methods		
			D	C	c	E	e	f	V	Cw	K	k	Kpa	Kpb	Jsa	Jsb	Fya	Fyb	Jka	Jkb	Lea	Leb	P1	M	N	S	s	LUa	LUb	Xga	37	AGH	CC
1	Bg(a+)	R1R1 B1080	+	+	0	0	+	0	0	0	0	+	0	+	0	+	+	0	0	+	0	+	+	+	+	+	+	0	+	+	1		
2		R1WR1 B1102	+	+	0	0	+	0	0	+	0	+	0	+	0	+	0	+	+	+	0	+	+	0	+	0	+	0	+	0	2		
3	Bg(a+)	R2R2 C1243	+	0	+	+	0	0	0	0	0	+	+	+	0	+	0	0	0	+	0	+	+	+	0	+	+	0	+	+	3		
4		ROR D575	+	0	+	0	+	+	0	0	0	+	+	+	0	+	0	0	+	0	0	0	+	+	+	0	+	0	+	+	4		
5		r'r E370	0	+	+	0	+	+	0	0	0	+	0	+	0	+	+	+	+	+	+	+	+	+	+	+	+	0	+	0	5		
6		r"r F416	0	0	+	+	+	+	0	0	0	+	0	+	0	+	0	+	+	+	+	0	+	+	+	0	+	+	+	+	6		
7		rrK G488	0	0	+	0	+	+	0	0	+	+	0	+	0	+	0	0	0	+	0	0	0	+	+	0	+	0	+	0	7		
8	Yt(b+)	rrFya H347	0	0	+	0	+	+	0	0	0	+	0	+	0	+	+	0	+	0	0	+	0	+	+	+	+	0	+	0	8		
9		rr N1434	0	0	+	0	+	+	0	0	0	+	0	+	0	+	+	+	+	0	+	0	+	0	+	+	+	0	+	+	9		
10	Co(b+)	R2R2 C199	+	0	+	+	0	0	0	0	0	+	0	+	0	+	+	+	+	0	+	0	+	+	+	0	+	0	+	+	10		
TC	He+	R1R2 A1086	+	+	+	+	+	0	0	0	0	+	0	+	0	+	0	0	0	+	0	+	+	+	+	+	+	+	+	0	TC		
		Patient's Cells																															

UNIVERSITY MEDICAL CENTER

Name: _____

Record #: _____

Date: _____

Time: _____

Cell Tests

Anti-A _____

Anti-B _____

Anti-D IS _____

Anti-D 37 _____

Anti-D AHG _____

Anti-A_1 Lectin _____

Serum Tests

	RT	37	AHG	CC
A_1 Cells	_____			
A_2 Cells	_____			
B Cells	_____			
Screen Cells I	_____	_____	_____	_____
Screen Cells II	_____	_____	_____	_____
Screen Cells III	_____	_____	_____	_____

UNIVERSITY MEDICAL CENTER
CONFIDENTIAL PATIENT INFORMATION
CUMULATIVE SUMMARY REPORT

PATIENT INFORMATION   ID number: _____   Ward: _____

Name: _____   Physician: _____

Address: _____   Date Admitted: _____

_____   Phone: _____

City: _____   State: _____   Zip: _____

Date of Birth: _____   Sex: _____   Race: _____

CHEMISTRY

Tests	Reference Ranges	Date: Time:	Date: Time:	Date: Time:	Date: Time:	Date: Time:
Acid Phos	2.5–11.7 U/L					
ACTH	9–52 pg/mL					
ALT	0–45 IU/L					
Albumin	3.5–5.0 g/dL					
A/G Ratio	0.7–2.1					
Aldosterone	??					
Alkaline Phos	41–137 IU/L					
Ammonia	11–35 μmol/L					
Amylase	95–290 U/L					
Anion Gap	10–18 mmol/L					
AST	0–41 IU/L					
Bilirubin	0.2–1.0 mg/dL					
Bilirubin (direct)	0.2–1.0 mg/dL					
BUN	10–20 mg/dL					
Calcium (total)	4.3–5.3 mEq/L					
Calcuim (ionized)	1.16–1.32 mmol/L					
Chloride	95–100 mmol/L					
Carbon Dioxide	23–32 mmol/L					

CHEMISTRY (page 2)						
Tests	Reference Ranges	Date: Time:	Date: Time:	Date: Time:	Date: Time:	Date: Time:
Cholesterol	<200 mg/dL					
CK	15–160 U/L					
CK-MB	15–160 U/L					
Creatinine	0.7–1.5 mg/dL					
Creatintine Clearance	80–120 mL/min					
GGT	6–45 U/L					
Globulin	2.3–3.2 g/dL					
Glucose	65–105 mg/dL					
LD	100–225 U/L					
LDL Cholesterol	75–140 U/L					
LDL/HDL	2.9–2.2					
Lipase	0–1.0 U/mL					
Magnesium	1.3–2.1 mEq/L					
Osmolality	275–295 mOsM/kg					
Phosphorus	2.7–4.5 mg/dL					
Potassium	3.5–5.0 mmol/L					
Protein	5.8–8.2 g/dL					
Sodium	135–145 mmol/L					
Triglycerides	10–190 mg/dL					
Uric Acid	3.5–7.2 mg/dL					
HCO_3	100–225 U/L					

PATIENT INFORMATION   ID number: _____   Ward: _____

Name: _____   Physician: _____

Address: _____   Date Admitted: _____

_____   Phone: _____

City: _____   State: _____   Zip: _____

Date of Birth: _____   Sex: _____   Race: _____

HEMATOLOGY

Test	Reference Ranges	Date: Time:	Date: Time:	Date: Time:	Date: Time:	Date: Time:
Hemoglobin (g/dL) Male Female	14.0–18.0 12.0–15.0					
Hematocrit (%) Male Female	40–54 35–49					
RBC ($\times 10^{12}$/L) Male Female	4.6–6.6 4.0–5.4					
WBC ($\times 10^{9}$/L)	4.5–11.5					
MCV (fL)	80–94					
MCHC (g/dL or %)	32–36					
MCH (pg)	26–32					
Platelet Count ($\times 10^{9}$/L)	150–450					
RDW (%)	11.5–14.5					
Reticulocyte Count						
Segmented Neutrophils (%)	50–70					
Lymphocytes (%)	18–42					
Monocytes (%)	2–11					
Basophils (%)	0–2					
Eosinophils (%)	1–3					
Erythrocyte Sed Rate (ESR) Male Female	0–9 mm/hr 0–15 mm/hr					
Prothrombin Time (PT)	<2-sec deviation from control; 12–14 sec					
Activated Partial Thromboplastin Time (APTT)	<35 sec					
Fibrin Degradation Products (FDP)	4.9 ± 2.8 µg FDP/mL					
Thrombin Time	15 sec					
D-Dimer	<0.5 µg/mL					

UNIVERSITY MEDICAL CENTER
CONFIDENTIAL PATIENT INFORMATION
CUMULATIVE SUMMARY REPORT

PATIENT INFORMATION   ID number: _____   Ward: _____

Name: _____   Physician: _____

Address: _____   Date Admitted: _____

_____   Phone: _____

City: _____   State: _____   Zip: _____

Date of Birth: _____   Sex: _____   Race: _____

MICROBIOLOGY

Date and Time	Procedure / Specimen	Direct Smear	Preliminary Report	Final Report

DIAGNOSIS 2

PATIENT INFORMATION

NAME: Michelle Craig   ID NUMBER: 37011

PHYSICIAN: Stark

DATE OF OFFICE VISIT: 8/7/96

ADDRESS: 354 Hodges, Chicago, IL 02425

PHONE: 000-555-3892

DATE OF BIRTH: 12/13/69   SEX: F   RACE: W

ADMISSION INFORMATION

WT.: 133 lb   HT.: 5'6"   B/P: 150/108

R: 20   PULSE: 90   TEMP.: 97.2

MEDICATION: Prednisone, Plaquenil

INITIAL DIAGNOSIS

Gastroenteritis

PRIMARY COMPLAINT

Diarrhea and vomiting; urinary urgency and burning

PATIENT HISTORY

Patient has been doing well until this past weekend, when she began diarrhea and vomiting. She suspects that she has eaten contaminated food and comes to the physician's office.

PROGRESS REPORTS

8/7/96: Patient was evaluated for routine laboratory tests and current status of her SLE. It was noted that she had 2+ pitting edema of the lower extremities. She was treated with Phenergan as needed and a clear liquid diet, and told to push fluids.

Treatment Plan:

Laboratory Tests Ordered: CBC, urinalysis, CMP, sedimentation rate, rheumatology profile, urine C&S

8/8/96: Patient was called and asked to return to the physician's office to follow up with a nephrology consult and additional laboratory studies in light of the results of the tests on 8/7.

8/9/96: Patient was seen at the Nephrology office to further assess her renal function.

Treatment Plan:

Laboratory Tests Ordered: Creatinine clearance, urinalysis, 24-h urine protein
Other Tests Ordered: Renal biopsy

8/14/96: Patient admitted to hospital; renal biopsy performed.

Results of Biopsy: The specimen consists of three pieces of pale tan tissue obtained from the right kidney. All glomeruli are involved and are membranous in appearance and proliferative with necrosis. Immunofluorescent stains are positive against IgA, IgG, C3, C4, and C1q. Fibrinogen, albumin, and properdin are negative. The striking finding is the presence of deposits in the glomerular basement membrane in an intramembranous distribution as well as a subendothelial distribution. Inflammatory cells are also seen. These findings are consistent with lupus nephritis.

8/16/96: Patient tolerated the renal biopsy well and was placed on oral Cytoxan. The patient's urinary tract infection was clearing, and her nausea and vomiting had resolved. It was felt that she had achieved maximal hospital benefit and could continue treatment and evaluation on an outpatient basis. Patient was discharged.

Treatment Plan:

Discharge Medications:
1. Prednisone
2. Plaquenil
3. Cytoxan
4. Floxin
5. Phenergan

Discharge Diagnosis:
1. Systemic lupus erythematosis
2. Nephritis secondary to lupus
3. Urinary tract infection
4. Nausea and vomiting

LEARNING ACTIVITIES

PATIENT: **Michelle Craig**
INSTRUCTIONS: *Before you begin, read the instructions carefully and follow each step in the process.*

STUDY GUIDES

Goal A

The goal in this activity is for you to relate laboratory data with Ms. Craig's symptoms, history, diagnosis, and prognosis on the initial office visit. This learning activity will allow you to collect and assess initial data pertaining to Ms. Craig during this presentation to her clinician.

Learning Issues

ISSUE 1: From the clinician's notes and Ms. Craig's progress reports, identify the clinical symtoms that helped the clinician in assessing the patient's condition.

ISSUE 2: Identify significant laboratory findings that are related to Ms. Craig's clinical condition during this admission. Correlate these findings with her clinical presentation.

ISSUE 3: Review the laboratory test results provided in the documentation and crrelate these data with Ms. Craig's diagnoses.

Study Questions

1. Review the patient's medical records and determine which of the presenting symptoms and which elements of the background history the physician may consider significant in her illness.

CLINICAL SYMPTOMS:

_____

_____

_____

_____

BACKGROUND HISTORY:

_____

_____

_____

_____

2. In the space provided, list the laboratory tests that were requested at the time of Ms. Craig's office visit on 8/7. Which of the tests requested specifically correlate with her presenting symptoms? Highlight these tests.

_____

_____

_____

_____

3. Now access the laboratory test results from the Laboratory Information System (LIS) in the CD-ROM. Obtain Ms. Craig's results and record them on the patient laboratory test results forms provided in this workbook. Review Ms. Craig's laboratory test results on 8/7.

4. Are any of the laboratory test results outside the normal acceptable range? List those results that are outside the normal acceptable range.

_____

_____

_____

_____

5. a. Are any of the lab results at critical levels?

_____

_____

_____

_____

   b. What do these results suggest?

_____

_____

_____

_____

6. Do these test results correlate with Ms. Craig's presenting symptoms? How?

7. As compared to January 1994, what is the status of Ms. Craig's anemia?

Goal B

In this portion of the learning activity, the goal is for you to evaluate follow-up measures taken during the course of Ms. Craig's illness and how these measures relate to her prognosis and ultimate outcome. This learning activity will allow you to identify reasons for the requests for additional laboratory tests to be performed on this patient.

Learning Issues

ISSUE 1: Interpret the data collected on Ms. Craig relating to treatment and prognosis.

ISSUE 2: Evaluate the use of the laboratory in this case.

Study Questions

1. As compared to January 1994, what is the status of Ms. Craig's SLE?

2. Which laboratory test results indicate renal function abnormalities?

3. What is the significance of a creatinine clearance evaluation?

4. How is a creatinine clearance test performed?

5. What is the formula for the calculation of creatinine clearance?

6. Explain the abnormal calcium and phosphorus results.

UNIVERSITY MEDICAL CENTER

Name: _____ Date: _____

Record #: _____ Time: _____

ANTIBODY IDENTIFICATION PANEL

Vial	Special Type	Donor	D	C	c	E	e	f	V	Cw	K	k	Kpa	Kpb	Jsa	Jsb	Fya	Fyb	Jka	Jkb	Lea	Leb	P1	M	N	S	s	LUa	LUb	Xga	37	AGH	CC	
						Rh-Hr							Kell				Duffy		Kidd		Lewis		P	MN				Lutheran		Xg	Test Methods			
1	Bg(a+)	R1R1 B1080	+	+	0	0	+	0	0	0	0	+	0	+	0	+	+	0	0	+	0	+	+	+	+	+	+	0	+	+				1
2		R1WR1 B1102	+	+	0	0	+	0	0	+	+	+	0	+	0	+	0	+	+	+	0	+	+	0	+	0	+	0	+	0				2
3	Bg(a+)	R2R2 C1243	+	0	+	+	0	0	0	0	0	+	0	+	0	+	+	+	0	0	0	+	+	+	0	+	+	0	+	+				3
4		ROR D575	+	0	+	0	+	+	0	0	0	+	0	+	0	+	0	0	+	0	0	0	+	0	+	0	+	0	+	+				4
5		r'r E370	0	+	+	0	+	+	0	0	0	+	0	+	0	+	+	+	0	+	0	+	+	+	+	+	+	0	+	0				5
6		r"r F416	0	0	+	+	+	+	0	0	0	+	0	+	0	+	0	+	+	+	+	0	0	+	0	0	+	+	+	+				6
7		rrK G488	0	0	+	0	+	+	0	0	+	+	0	+	0	+	0	0	0	0	+	0	0	+	0	0	+	0	+	0				7
8	Yt(b+)	rrFya H347	0	0	+	0	+	+	0	0	0	+	0	+	0	+	+	+	+	0	0	+	+	+	0	+	+	0	+	0				8
9		rr N1434	0	0	+	0	+	+	0	0	0	+	0	+	0	+	+	+	0	0	0	+	+	+	+	+	0	0	+	+				9
10	Co(b+)	R2R2 C199	+	0	+	+	0	0	0	0	0	+	0	+	0	+	+	+	+	0	+	0	+	+	+	0	+	0	+	+				10
TC	He+	R1R2 A1086	+	+	+	+	+	0	0	0	0	+	0	+	0	+	0	0	0	+	0	+	+	+	+	+	+	+	+	0				TC
		Patient's Cells																																

UNIVERSITY MEDICAL CENTER

Name: _____

Date: _____

Record #: _____

Time: _____

Cell Tests

Anti-A _____

Anti-B _____

Anti-D IS _____

Anti-D 37 _____

Anti-D AHG _____

Anti-A_1 Lectin _____

Serum Tests

A_1 Cells _____

A_2 Cells _____

B Cells _____

	RT	37	AHG	CC
Screen Cells I	___	___	___	___
Screen Cells II	___	___	___	___
Screen Cells III	___	___	___	___

UNIVERSITY MEDICAL CENTER
CONFIDENTIAL PATIENT INFORMATION
CUMULATIVE SUMMARY REPORT

PATIENT INFORMATION   ID number: _____   Ward: _____

Name: _____   Physician: _____

Address: _____   Date Admitted: _____

_____   Phone: _____

City: _____   State: _____   Zip: _____

Date of Birth: _____   Sex: _____   Race: _____

CHEMISTRY

Tests	Reference Ranges	Date: Time:	Date: Time:	Date: Time:	Date: Time:	Date: Time:
Acid Phos	2.5–11.7 U/L					
ACTH	9–52 pg/mL					
ALT	0–45 IU/L					
Albumin	3.5–5.0 g/dL					
A/G Ratio	0.7–2.1					
Aldosterone	??					
Alkaline Phos	41–137 IU/L					
Ammonia	11–35 µmol/L					
Amylase	95–290 U/L					
Anion Gap	10–18 mmol/L					
AST	0–41 IU/L					
Bilirubin	0.2–1.0 mg/dL					
Bilirubin (direct)	0.2–1.0 mg/dL					
BUN	10–20 mg/dL					
Calcium (total)	4.3–5.3 mEq/L					
Calcuim (ionized)	1.16–1.32 mmol/L					
Chloride	95–100 mmol/L					
Carbon Dioxide	23–32 mmol/L					

CHEMISTRY (page 2)

Tests	Reference Ranges	Date: Time:	Date: Time:	Date: Time:	Date: Time:	Date: Time:
Cholesterol	<200 mg/dL					
CK	15–160 U/L					
CK-MB	15–160 U/L					
Creatinine	0.7–1.5 mg/dL					
Creatintine Clearance	80–120 mL/min					
GGT	6–45 U/L					
Globulin	2.3–3.2 g/dL					
Glucose	65–105 mg/dL					
LD	100–225 U/L					
LDL Cholesterol	75–140 U/L					
LDL/HDL	2.9–2.2					
Lipase	0–1.0 U/mL					
Magnesium	1.3–2.1 mEq/L					
Osmolality	275–295 mOsM/kg					
Phosphorus	2.7–4.5 mg/dL					
Potassium	3.5–5.0 mmol/L					
Protein	5.8–8.2 g/dL					
Sodium	135–145 mmol/L					
Triglycerides	10–190 mg/dL					
Uric Acid	3.5–7.2 mg/dL					
HCO_3	100–225 U/L					

CONFIDENTIAL PATIENT INFORMATION
CUMULATIVE SUMMARY REPORT

PATIENT INFORMATION   ID number: _____   Ward: _____

Name: _____   Physician: _____

Address: _____   Date Admitted: _____

_____   Phone: _____

City: _____   State: _____   Zip: _____

Date of Birth: _____   Sex: _____   Race: _____

HEMATOLOGY

Test	Reference Ranges	Date: Time:	Date: Time:	Date: Time:	Date: Time:	Date: Time:
Hemoglobin (g/dL) Male Female	14.0–18.0 12.0–15.0					
Hematocrit (%) Male Female	40–54 35–49					
RBC ($\times 10^{12}$/L) Male Female	4.6–6.6 4.0–5.4					
WBC ($\times 10^{9}$/L)	4.5–11.5					
MCV (fL)	80–94					
MCHC (g/dL or %)	32–36					
MCH (pg)	26–32					
Platelet Count ($\times 10^{9}$/L)	150–450					
RDW (%)	11.5–14.5					
Reticulocyte Count						
Segmented Neutrophils (%)	50–70					
Lymphocytes (%)	18–42					
Monocytes (%)	2–11					
Basophils (%)	0–2					
Eosinophils (%)	1–3					
Erythrocyte Sed Rate (ESR) Male Female	0–9 mm/hr 0–15 mm/hr					
Prothrombin Time (PT)	<2-sec deviation from control; 12–14 sec					
Activated Partial Thromboplastin Time (APTT)	<35 sec					
Fibrin Degradation Products (FDP)	4.9 ± 2.8 µg FDP/mL					
Thrombin Time	15 sec					
D-Dimer	<0.5 µg/mL					

UNIVERSITY MEDICAL CENTER

CONFIDENTIAL PATIENT INFORMATION
CUMULATIVE SUMMARY REPORT

PATIENT INFORMATION   ID number: _____   Ward: _____

Name: _____   Physician: _____

Address: _____   Date Admitted: _____

_____   Phone: _____

City: _____   State: _____   Zip: _____

Date of Birth: _____   Sex: _____   Race: _____

MICROBIOLOGY

Date and Time	Procedure / Specimen	Direct Smear	Preliminary Report	Final Report

DIAGNOSIS 3

PATIENT INFORMATION

NAME: Michelle Craig   ID NUMBER: 37011

PHYSICIAN: Stark

DATE OF OFFICE VISIT: 7/23/98

ADDRESS: 354 Hodges, Chicago, IL 02425

PHONE: 000-555-3892

DATE OF BIRTH: 12/13/69   SEX: F   RACE: W

ADMISSION INFORMATION

WT.: 120   HT.: 5'6"   B/P: 130/72

R: 16   PULSE: 88   TEMP.: 98.2

MEDICATION: Prednisone, Plaquenil, Cytoxan

ADMISSION DIAGNOSIS

SLE, lupus nephritis

PRIMARY COMPLAINT

Weak, shaky, no appetite, nausea

PATIENT HISTORY

Patient states that she has been feeling weak for about 1 week. She has had a cough, a mild postnasal drip, and sweats. She is concerned that she is having a recurrence of her lupus. She has not been having arthralgias, skin rash, photosensitivity, mouth ulcers, hair loss, or any other symptoms beyond those stated here. She has had anemia associated with her lupus previously. She is having a sensation of rapid heartbeats.

TREATMENT PLAN

Laboratory Tests Ordered: CMP, CBC, sedimentation rate, UA, CRP, rheumatology profile, ECG

PROGRESS REPORTS

7/23/98: Assessment; laboratory reports are reviewed.

Treatment Plan: Patient placed on antibiotics and advised to return for checkup in 2 weeks.

8/3/98: Patient returns with continuing symptoms and increasing nausea and fatigue. Review of testing for lupus indicates that this is not a flare-up of lupus. Investigate other viral conditions. Recheck in 1 week.

Treatment Plan:

Laboratory Tests Ordered: CBC, UA, CMP, iron profile, thyroid profile, CMV, EBV, liver profile, hepatitis profile

8/11/98: Patient returns to discuss results of laboratory testing of 8/3. No significant changes on CBC, UA, and CMP. Begin treatment with propylthiouracil (PTU), 50 mg QID. Will check thyroid antibodies.

Treatment Plan:

Laboratory Tests Ordered: Thyroid-stimulating immunoglobulins

8/26/98:

Follow-up of Patient: Patient is feeling much better, with greater energy and much less nausea. Laboratory results reflect a normalizing T4 but a worsening anemia. Continue PTU and treat anemia with iron and multivitamin supplements.

Treatment Plan:

Laboratory Tests Ordered: CBC, thyroid profile

9/10/98:

Follow-up of Hyperthyroidism: Patient is feeling much better, and laboratory results are normal. Continue medications as indicated.

Treatment Plan:

Laboratory Tests Ordered: Thyroid profile, CBC

A period of approximately 16 months passes, during which time Ms. Craig remains euthyroid and slightly anemic.

1/28/00: Patient returns for routine office visit and complains of fatigue. Laboratory results show abnormalities consistent with hyperthyroidism and a more severe anemia. Schedule appointment in 1 month to check condition.

Treatment Plan:

Laboratory Tests Ordered: CBC, thyroid profile

2/28/00: Patient has no additional complaints, but there is laboratory evidence of deteriorating anemia and increasing hyperthyroidism. Patient told to discontinue PTU due to depression of the bone marrow.

Treatment Plan:

Laboratory Tests Ordered: CBC, thyroid profile
Other Tests Ordered: Radioactive iodine (RAI) uptake

3/13/00: Ms. Craig's radioactive iodine results indicate that she is a good candidate for RAI therapy.

Treatment Plan: Schedule for RAI therapy 3/15/00.

4/18/00: Ms. Craig returns for evaluation of thyroid status. She states that she is feeling better and is gaining some weight.

Treatment Plan:

Laboratory Tests Ordered: Thyroid profile

6/14/00: Ms. Craig returns for follow-up of thyroid status. She complains that she is weak and easily fatigued.

Treatment Plan:

Laboratory Tests Ordered: Thyroid profile, CBC
        Place the patient on Synthroid.

LEARNING ACTIVITIES

PATIENT: Michelle Craig
INSTRUCTIONS: *Before you begin, read the instructions carefully and follow each step in the process.*

STUDY GUIDES

Goal A

The goal in this activity is for you to relate laboratory data with Ms. Craig's symptoms, history, diagnosis, and prognosis on these office visits. This learning activity will allow you to collect and assess initial data pertaining to Ms. Craig.

Learning Issues

ISSUE 1: From the clinician's notes and Ms. Craig's progress reports, identify the clinical symptoms that helped the clinician in assessing the patient's condition during her visit to the physician's office.

ISSUE 2: Identify significant laboratory findings that are related to Ms. Craig's clinical condition during the follow-up visits. Correlate these findings with her clinical presentation.

Issue 3: Review the laboratory test results provided in the documentation and correlate these data with Ms. Craig's prognosis.

Study Questions A

1. Review the patient's medical records and determine which of the presenting symptoms and which elements of the background history the physician may consider significant in her illness.

CLINICAL SYMPTOMS:

BACKGROUND HISTORY:

2. In the space provided, list the laboratory tests that were requested at the time of Ms. Craig's initial office visit. Which of the tests requested specifically correlate with her presenting symptoms? Highlight these tests.

3. Now access the laboratory test results from the Laboratory Information System (LIS) in the CD-ROM. Obtain Ms. Craig's results and record them on the patient laboratory test results forms provided in this workbook. Review Ms. Craig's laboratory test results on 7/23/98.

4. a. Are any of the laboratory test results outside the normal acceptable ranges? List those results that are outside the normal acceptable ranges.

   b. Which lab results indicate a renal problem?

5. a. Are any lab results at critical levels?

   b. What do these results suggest?

   c. Do these test results correlate with Ms. Craig's presenting symptoms? How?

6. Are Ms. Craig's symptoms reflective of a thyroid problem? If so, which one(s)?

7. How are we able to determine if Ms. Craig's hyperthyroidism is primary or secondary?

8. Which autoantibodies are commonly found in patients with Graves' disease?

Goal B

In this portion of the learning activity, the goal is for you to evaluate follow-up measures taken during the course of Ms. Craig's illness and how these measures relate to her prognosis and ultimate outcome. This learning activity will allow you to identify reasons for the requests for additional laboratory tests to be performed on this patient.

Learning Issues

ISSUE 1: Interpret the data collected on Ms. Craig relating to treatment and prognosis.

ISSUE 2: Evaluate the use of the laboratory in this case.

Study Questions B

1. Ms. Craig was initially treated with medication to reduce the production of thyroid hormones. When this medication complicated her anemia, it was discontinued and radioactive iodine treatment was used to destroy thyroid cells. After 3 months, Ms. Craig became hypothyroid. Is this a common occurrence, and were there alternative treatments that might have prevented Ms. Craig's hypothyroidism?

2. Is there a common pathology that links Ms. Craig's three diagnoses? If so, what is it?

3. Are there any laboratory tests that have not been ordered on Ms. Craig that would be helpful in arriving at a more specific diagnosis? If so, what tests do you think were omitted?

4. Discuss the appropriateness of the laboratory tests ordered on Ms. Craig. Is the laboratory being overutilized or underutilized? Defend your answer.

Name: _____   Date: _____

Record #: _____   Time: _____

ANTIBODY IDENTIFICATION PANEL

Vial	Special Type	Donor	D	C	c	E	e	f	V	Cw	K	k	Kpa	Kpb	Jsa	Jsb	Fya	Fyb	Jka	Jkb	Lea	Leb	P1	M	N	S	s	LUa	LUb	Xga	37	AGH	CC	
1	Bg(a+)	R1R1 B1080	+	+	0	0	+	0	0	0	0	+	0	+	0	+	+	0	0	+	0	+	+	+	+	+	+	0	+	+				1
2		R1WR1 B1102	+	+	0	0	0	0	0	+	+	+	0	+	0	+	0	+	+	+	0	+	+	0	+	0	+	0	+	0				2
3	Bg(a+)	R2R2 C1243	+	0	+	+	0	0	0	0	0	+	0	+	0	+	+	+	0	+	0	+	+	+	0	+	+	0	+	+				3
4		ROR D575	+	0	+	0	+	+	0	0	0	+	0	+	0	+	0	0	+	0	0	0	+	0	+	0	+	0	+	+				4
5		r'r E370	0	+	+	0	+	+	0	0	0	+	0	+	0	+	+	+	+	+	+	0	+	+	+	+	+	0	+	0				5
6		r"r F416	0	0	+	+	+	+	0	0	0	+	0	+	0	+	+	+	0	+	0	+	0	+	+	0	+	+	+	+				6
7		rrK G488	0	0	+	0	+	+	0	0	+	+	0	+	0	+	+	0	+	0	+	0	0	+	0	0	+	0	+	0				7
8	Yt(b+)	rrFya H347	0	0	+	0	+	+	0	0	0	+	0	+	0	+	0	+	+	+	+	0	+	+	+	+	+	0	+	0				8
9		rr N1434	0	0	+	0	+	+	0	0	0	+	0	+	0	+	+	0	0	+	0	+	+	0	+	0	0	0	+	+				9
10	Co(b+)	R2R2 C199	+	0	+	+	0	0	0	0	0	+	0	+	0	+	+	+	+	0	0	0	0	+	+	0	+	0	+	+				10
TC	He+	R1R2 A1086	+	+	+	+	+	0	0	0	0	+	0	+	0	+	0	0	0	+	0	+	+	+	+	+	+	+	+	0				TC
		Patient's Cells																																

UNIVERSITY MEDICAL CENTER

Name: _____

Record #: _____

Date: _____

Time: _____

Cell Tests

Anti-A _____

Anti-B _____

Anti-D IS _____

Anti-D 37 _____

Anti-D AHG _____

Anti-A$_1$ Lectin _____

Serum Tests

	RT	37	AHG	CC
A$_1$ Cells	___			
A$_2$ Cells	___			
B Cells	___			
Screen Cells I	___	___	___	___
Screen Cells II	___	___	___	___
Screen Cells III	___	___	___	___

UNIVERSITY MEDICAL CENTER
CONFIDENTIAL PATIENT INFORMATION
CUMULATIVE SUMMARY REPORT

PATIENT INFORMATION   ID number: _____   Ward: _____

Name: _____   Physician: _____

Address: _____   Date Admitted: _____

_____   Phone: _____

City: _____   State: _____   Zip: _____

Date of Birth: _____   Sex: _____   Race: _____

CHEMISTRY

Tests	Reference Ranges	Date: Time:	Date: Time:	Date: Time:	Date: Time:	Date: Time:
Acid Phos	2.5–11.7 U/L					
ACTH	9–52 pg/mL					
ALT	0–45 IU/L					
Albumin	3.5–5.0 g/dL					
A/G Ratio	0.7–2.1					
Aldosterone	??					
Alkaline Phos	41–137 IU/L					
Ammonia	11–35 μmol/L					
Amylase	95–290 U/L					
Anion Gap	10–18 mmol/L					
AST	0–41 IU/L					
Bilirubin	0.2–1.0 mg/dL					
Bilirubin (direct)	0.2–1.0 mg/dL					
BUN	10–20 mg/dL					
Calcium (total)	4.3–5.3 mEq/L					
Calcuim (ionized)	1.16–1.32 mmol/L					
Chloride	95–100 mmol/L					
Carbon Dioxide	23–32 mmol/L					

CHEMISTRY (page 2)

Tests	Reference Ranges	Date: Time:	Date: Time:	Date: Time:	Date: Time:	Date: Time:
Cholesterol	<200 mg/dL					
CK	15–160 U/L					
CK-MB	15–160 U/L					
Creatinine	0.7–1.5 mg/dL					
Creatintine Clearance	80–120 mL/min					
GGT	6–45 U/L					
Globulin	2.3–3.2 g/dL					
Glucose	65–105 mg/dL					
LD	100–225 U/L					
LDL Cholesterol	75–140 U/L					
LDL/HDL	2.9–2.2					
Lipase	0–1.0 U/mL					
Magnesium	1.3–2.1 mEq/L					
Osmolality	275–295 mOsM/kg					
Phosphorus	2.7–4.5 mg/dL					
Potassium	3.5–5.0 mmol/L					
Protein	5.8–8.2 g/dL					
Sodium	135–145 mmol/L					
Triglycerides	10–190 mg/dL					
Uric Acid	3.5–7.2 mg/dL					
HCO_3	100–225 U/L					

UNIVERSITY MEDICAL CENTER
CONFIDENTIAL PATIENT INFORMATION
CUMULATIVE SUMMARY REPORT

PATIENT INFORMATION   ID number: _____   Ward: _____

Name: _____   Physician: _____

Address: _____   Date Admitted: _____

_____   Phone: _____

City: _____   State: _____   Zip: _____

Date of Birth: _____   Sex: _____   Race: _____

HEMATOLOGY

Test	Reference Ranges	Date: Time:	Date: Time:	Date: Time:	Date: Time:	Date: Time:
Hemoglobin (g/dL) Male Female	14.0–18.0 12.0–15.0					
Hematocrit (%) Male Female	40–54 35–49					
RBC ($\times 10^{12}$/L) Male Female	4.6–6.6 4.0–5.4					
WBC ($\times 10^9$/L)	4.5–11.5					
MCV (fL)	80–94					
MCHC (g/dL or %)	32–36					
MCH (pg)	26–32					
Platelet Count ($\times 10^9$/L)	150–450					
RDW (%)	11.5–14.5					
Reticulocyte Count						
Segmented Neutrophils (%)	50–70					
Lymphocytes (%)	18–42					
Monocytes (%)	2–11					
Basophils (%)	0–2					
Eosinophils (%)	1–3					
Erythrocyte Sed Rate (ESR) Male Female	0–9 mm/hr 0–15 mm/hr					
Prothrombin Time (PT)	<2-sec deviation from control; 12–14 sec					
Activated Partial Thromboplastin Time (APTT)	<35 sec					
Fibrin Degradation Products (FDP)	4.9 ± 2.8 µg FDP/mL					
Thrombin Time	15 sec					
D-Dimer	<0.5 µg/mL					

UNIVERSITY MEDICAL CENTER

CONFIDENTIAL PATIENT INFORMATION
CUMULATIVE SUMMARY REPORT

PATIENT INFORMATION   ID number: _____   Ward: _____

Name: _____   Physician: _____

Address: _____   Date Admitted: _____

_____   Phone: _____

City: _____   State: _____   Zip: _____

Date of Birth: _____   Sex: _____   Race: _____

MICROBIOLOGY

Date and Time	Procedure / Specimen	Direct Smear	Preliminary Report	Final Report

CASE SUMMARY

A. Provide a brief summary of possible patient outcomes based on the laboratory test results and the patient's diagnoses.

B. Identify the learning points that you consider helpful in working up this patient's case. *(This will be an individual response.)*

NOTES

► PATIENT'S RECORDS

PATIENT NAME: **Kenya Fielder**

PATIENT IDENTIFICATION NUMBER: **691350**

PHYSICIAN: **Brown**

PATIENT INFORMATION

NAME: Kenya Fielder   ID NUMBER: 691350

PHYSICIAN: Brown

DATE ADMITTED: 12/03/02   TIME: 1940

ADDRESS: 7373 Old Wagon Tr., Milwaukee, WI 09222

PHONE: 000-455-4455

DATE OF BIRTH: 09/05/37   SEX: F   RACE: B

ADMISSION INFORMATION

WT.: 135 lb   HT.: 5'10"   B/P: 158/94

R: 17   PULSE: 88   TEMP.: 97.3

MEDICATION: None

ADMISSION DIAGNOSIS

Splenomegaly

PRIMARY COMPLAINT

Abdominal pain; shortness of breath

PATIENT HISTORY

The patient, a 65-year-old African American female, was admitted to the hospital 2 days ago with complaints of abdominal pain and shortness of breath. The diagnosis of splenomegaly caused by hereditary elliptocytosis was made by the physician. Since the patient is experiencing an uncompensated hemolytic anemia, a splenectomy has been scheduled. The patient has had three children. She received 2 units of red blood cells 40 years ago following the birth of her third child. She hasn't been to any hospital since. This is her first visit to this hospital. She is currently taking no prescription medications.

TREATMENT PLAN

Schedule patient for surgery to remove the patient's spleen. Four units of red blood cells are ordered if needed during or following surgery.
Laboratory Tests Ordered: CBC, electrolytes, PT, APTT, UA

PROGRESS REPORTS

12/05/02, 1000: Patient was taken to surgery to remove spleen.

Treatment Plan:

Laboratory Tests Ordered: Hemoglobin and hematocrit twice daily

12/05/02, 1800: Patient's hemoglobin and hematocrit remain low.

Treatment Plan: Transfuse 2 units of packed red blood cells. Hemoglobin and hematocrit in the A.M.

12/06/02, 0800: Patient is stable. No complications from surgery.

Treatment Plan: Hemoglobin and hematocrit in the a.m. Plan for discharge. Follow up as outpatient in 10 days.

LEARNING ACTIVITIES

PATIENT: Kenya Fielder
INSTRUCTIONS: *Before you begin, read the instructions carefully and follow each stip in the process.*

STUDY GUIDES

Goal A

The goal in this activity is for you to relate laboratory data with Ms. Fielder's symptoms on her admission to the hospital. This learning activity will allow you to collect and assess initial data pertaining to Ms. Fielder.

Learning Issues

ISSUE 1: From the clinician's notes, identify relevant signs and symptoms, social and previous medical history, and results of the physical examination.

ISSUE 2: Identify significant laboratory findings that are related to Ms. Fielder's clinical condition at the time of presentation. Correlate these findings with her clinical presentation.

ISSUE 3: Review the laboratory test results provided in the documentation and identify discrepancies, if any, that may need to be resolved.

Study Questions A

1. Review the patient's medical records and determine which of the presenting symptoms and which elements of the background history the physician may consider significant in her illness.

CLINICAL SYMPTOMS:

BACKGROUND HISTORY:

2. In the space provided, list the laboratory tests that were requested at the time of Ms. Fielder's admission to the facility. Which of the tests requested specifically correlate with her presenting symptoms? Highlight these tests.

3. Now access the laboratory test results from the Laboratory Information System (LIS) in the CD-ROM. Obtain Ms. Fielder's laboratory results on admission and record them on the patient laboratory test results forms provided in this workbook. Review Ms. Fielder's laboratory test results at the time she was admitted to the hospital.

Note: If this is your first time accessing information in the CD-ROM, make sure that you start with "Before you begin."

4. a. Are any of the laboratory test results outside the usual acceptable range? List those results that are outside the usual acceptable range.

b. What do these results indicate?

Goal B

In this portion of the learning activity, the goal is for you to evaluate follow-up measures taken regarding Ms. Fielder's condition. This learning activity will allow you to identify discrepancies in laboratory test results and understand how these issues are resolved with additional testing if needed.

Learning Issues

ISSUE 1: Interpret the data obtained and provide the appropriate blood product(s) for this patient.

ISSUE 2: Evaluate the use of the laboratory in this case.

1. Access the blood bank test results from the LIS in the CD-ROM. Obtain Ms. Fielder's blood bank results and record them on the blood bank results form provided in this workbook. Review the test results and the interpretation of the results provided.

2. What is the patient's ABO/Rh group?

    _____

    _____

    _____

    _____

3. Review the compatibility test results.

    a. Are there any incompatibilities observed? What could be the cause
    of these test results?

    _____

    _____

    _____

    _____

    b. What test should be performed on the unit that showed an incom-
    patibility to reveal the cause of this result?

    _____

    _____

    _____

    _____

    c. What could be the cause of the 4+ result in the compatibility test
    with unit 12158?

    _____

    _____

    _____

    _____

    d. What could be the reason for the mislabeling of this unit?

    _____

    _____

    _____

    _____

4. What red blood cell products should you provide for this patient?

5. What could be the results of the investigation of the mislabeling of this unit?

6. What is the most common severe form of transfusion reaction, and what is the usual cause of such a transfusion reaction?

Name: _____ Date: _____

Record #: _____ Time: _____

ANTIBODY IDENTIFICATION PANEL

Vial	Special Type	Donor	Rh-Hr								Kell						Duffy		Kidd		Lewis		P	MN				Lutheran		Xg	Test Methods			
			D	C	c	E	e	f	V	Cw	K	k	Kp_a	Kp_b	Js_a	Js_b	Fy_a	Fy_b	Jk_a	Jk_b	Le_a	Le_b	P1	M	N	S	s	LU_a	LU_b	Xg_a		37	AGH	CC
1	Bg(a+)	R1R1 B1080	+	+	0	0	+	0	0	0	0	+	0	+	0	+	+	0	0	+	0	+	+	+	+	+	+	0	+	+	1			
2		R1WR1 B1102	+	+	0	0	+	0	0	+	0	+	0	+	0	+	0	+	+	+	0	+	+	0	+	0	+	0	+	0	2			
3	Bg(a+)	R2R2 C1243	+	0	+	+	0	0	0	0	0	+	0	+	0	+	+	+	0	+	0	+	+	+	0	+	+	0	+	+	3			
4		ROR D575	+	0	+	0	+	+	0	0	0	+	0	+	0	+	0	+	+	0	0	0	+	0	+	0	+	0	+	+	4			
5		r'r E370	0	+	+	0	+	+	0	0	0	+	0	+	0	+	+	+	0	0	0	0	+	+	+	+	+	0	+	0	5			
6		r"r F416	0	0	+	+	+	+	0	0	0	+	0	+	0	+	0	+	+	+	+	0	0	+	0	0	+	+	+	+	6			
7		rrK G488	0	0	+	0	+	+	0	0	+	0	0	+	0	+	0	+	0	+	0	0	0	+	0	0	+	0	+	0	7			
8	Yt(b+)	rrFya H347	0	0	+	0	+	+	0	0	0	+	0	+	0	+	+	0	+	+	0	+	+	+	0	+	+	0	+	0	8			
9		rr N1434	0	0	+	0	+	+	0	0	0	+	0	+	0	+	+	+	+	+	0	+	+	+	0	+	0	0	+	+	9			
10	Co(b+)	R2R2 C199	+	0	+	+	0	0	0	0	0	+	0	+	0	+	+	0	+	0	+	0	+	+	+	0	+	0	+	+	10			
TC	He+	R1R2 A1086	+	+	+	+	+	+	0	0	0	+	0	+	0	+	0	+	0	+	0	+	+	+	+	+	+	+	+	0	TC			
		Patient's Cells																																	

UNIVERSITY MEDICAL CENTER

Name: _____

Record #: _____

Date: _____

Time: _____

Cell Tests

Anti-A _____

Anti-B _____

Anti-D IS _____

Anti-D 37 _____

Anti-D AHG _____

Anti-A₁ Lectin _____

Serum Tests

	RT	37	AHG	CC
A₁ Cells	_____			
A₂ Cells	_____			
B Cells	_____			
Screen Cells I	_____	_____	_____	_____
Screen Cells II	_____	_____	_____	_____
Screen Cells III	_____	_____	_____	_____

UNIVERSITY MEDICAL CENTER
CONFIDENTIAL PATIENT INFORMATION
CUMULATIVE SUMMARY REPORT

PATIENT INFORMATION   ID number: _____   Ward: _____

Name: _____   Physician: _____

Address: _____   Date Admitted: _____

_____   Phone: _____

City: _____   State: _____   Zip: _____

Date of Birth: _____   Sex: _____   Race: _____

CHEMISTRY

Tests	Reference Ranges	Date: Time:	Date: Time:	Date: Time:	Date: Time:	Date: Time:
Acid Phos	2.5–11.7 U/L					
ACTH	9–52 pg/mL					
ALT	0–45 IU/L					
Albumin	3.5–5.0 g/dL					
A/G Ratio	0.7–2.1					
Aldosterone	??					
Alkaline Phos	41–137 IU/L					
Ammonia	11–35 µmol/L					
Amylase	95–290 U/L					
Anion Gap	10–18 mmol/L					
AST	0–41 IU/L					
Bilirubin	0.2–1.0 mg/dL					
Bilirubin (direct)	0.2–1.0 mg/dL					
BUN	10–20 mg/dL					
Calcium (total)	4.3–5.3 mEq/L					
Calcuim (ionized)	1.16–1.32 mmol/L					
Chloride	95–100 mmol/L					
Carbon Dioxide	23–32 mmol/L					

CHEMISTRY (page 2)

Tests	Reference Ranges	Date: Time:	Date: Time:	Date: Time:	Date: Time:	Date: Time:
Cholesterol	<200 mg/dL					
CK	15–160 U/L					
CK-MB	15–160 U/L					
Creatinine	0.7–1.5 mg/dL					
Creatintine Clearance	80–120 mL/min					
GGT	6–45 U/L					
Globulin	2.3–3.2 g/dL					
Glucose	65–105 mg/dL					
LD	100–225 U/L					
LDL Cholesterol	75–140 U/L					
LDL/HDL	2.9–2.2					
Lipase	0–1.0 U/mL					
Magnesium	1.3–2.1 mEq/L					
Osmolality	275–295 mOsM/kg					
Phosphorus	2.7–4.5 mg/dL					
Potassium	3.5–5.0 mmol/L					
Protein	5.8–8.2 g/dL					
Sodium	135–145 mmol/L					
Triglycerides	10–190 mg/dL					
Uric Acid	3.5–7.2 mg/dL					
HCO_3	100–225 U/L					

UNIVERSITY MEDICAL CENTER
CONFIDENTIAL PATIENT INFORMATION
CUMULATIVE SUMMARY REPORT

PATIENT INFORMATION   ID number: _____   Ward: _____

Name: _____   Physician: _____

Address: _____   Date Admitted: _____

_____   Phone: _____

City: _____   State: _____   Zip: _____

Date of Birth: _____   Sex: _____   Race: _____

HEMATOLOGY

Test	Reference Ranges	Date: Time:	Date: Time:	Date: Time:	Date: Time:	Date: Time:
Hemoglobin (g/dL) Male Female	14.0–18.0 12.0–15.0					
Hematocrit (%) Male Female	40–54 35–49					
RBC ($\times 10^{12}$/L) Male Female	4.6–6.6 4.0–5.4					
WBC ($\times 10^{9}$/L)	4.5–11.5					
MCV (fL)	80–94					
MCHC (g/dL or %)	32–36					
MCH (pg)	26–32					
Platelet Count ($\times 10^{9}$/L)	150–450					
RDW (%)	11.5–14.5					
Reticulocyte Count						
Segmented Neutrophils (%)	50–70					
Lymphocytes (%)	18–42					
Monocytes (%)	2–11					
Basophils (%)	0–2					
Eosinophils (%)	1–3					
Erythrocyte Sed Rate (ESR) Male Female	0–9 mm/hr 0–15 mm/hr					
Prothrombin Time (PT)	<2-sec deviation from control; 12–14 sec					
Activated Partial Thromboplastin Time (APTT)	<35 sec					
Fibrin Degradation Products (FDP)	4.9 ± 2.8 µg FDP/mL					
Thrombin Time	15 sec					
D-Dimer	<0.5 µg/mL					

UNIVERSITY MEDICAL CENTER
CONFIDENTIAL PATIENT INFORMATION
CUMULATIVE SUMMARY REPORT

PATIENT INFORMATION   ID number: _____   Ward: _____

Name: _____   Physician: _____

Address: _____   Date Admitted: _____

_____   Phone: _____

City: _____   State: _____   Zip: _____

Date of Birth: _____   Sex: _____   Race: _____

MICROBIOLOGY

Date and Time	Procedure / Specimen	Direct Smear	Preliminary Report	Final Report

CASE SUMMARY

A. Provide a brief summary of possible patient outcomes based on the laboratory test results and the patient's diagnoses.

B. Identify the learning points that you consider helpful in working up this patient's case. *(This will be an individual response.)*

NOTES

► PATIENT'S RECORDS

PATIENT NAME: **Alfred Gates**

PATIENT IDENTIFICATION NUMBER: **212011**

PHYSICIAN: **Roman**

PATIENT INFORMATION

NAME: Alfred Gates   ID NUMBER: 212011

PHYSICIAN: Roman

DATE ADMITTED: 01/15/02   TIME: 1300

ADDRESS: 100 Central Ave., Ivanville, ID 13012

PHONE: 200-555-1212

DATE OF BIRTH: 03/15/46   SEX: M   RACE: W   WARD: 3S

ADMISSION INFORMATION

WT.: 130 lb   HT.: 6'1"   B/P: 130/80

R: 24   PULSE: 110   TEMP.: 101.2

ADMISSION DIAGNOSIS
Fever of unknown origin

PRIMARY COMPLAINT
Fever, fatigue, pain in right groin

PATIENT HISTORY
The patient is a 56-year-old white male who has experienced chronic fatigue and fever for the past 4 weeks. He also complains of pain in his right groin.

The patient has a history of smoking two packs of cigarettes per day for 6 to 7 years. He reports occasional consumption of alcohol and no drug usage. The family history shows no evidence of malignancies; however, a number of family members have died from coronary artery disease.

PHYSICAL EXAMINATION

The patient showed right inguinal lymphadenopathy and tenderness of the abdomen, appeared weak, and was febrile.

TREATMENT PLAN

CT scan of abdomen and chest

Laboratory Tests Ordered: Tissue biopsy of lymph node in the right groin, CBC

PROGRESS REPORTS

1/18/02, 1800: Patient remained stable. Fever persisted. Loss of appetite.

CT scan of the chest showed mediastinal lymphadenopathy. CT scan of the abdomen showed splenomegaly.

Initial Diagnosis: Anemia, leukemia

Treatment Plan: Request bone marrow biopsy. Request flow cytometry studies.

1/19/02, 1000: Biopsy of the inguinal lymph nodes and bone marrow studies determined final diagnosis.

Treatment Plan: Start chemotherapy. Transfuse 3 units of packed red blood cells and 8 units of platelet concentrates.

1/20/02, 0600: The patient remained stable.

Treatment Plan: Continue chemotherapy and follow-up treatment in the outpatient clinic.

4/25/02: Abscess formed in the groin region.

Treatment Plan: Discontinue cytarabine.

5/15/02: Patient presented at the clinic with small preauricular nodes. Indicative of recurrence.

Treatment Plan: Restart chemotherapy. Order biopsy of bone marrow.

6/25/02: The patient completed chemotherapy. Results of bone marrow biopsy showed no lymphoma.

Treatment Plan: Schedule for autologous bone marrow transplant.

8/09/02: The patient developed fever.

Treatment Plan:

Laboratory Tests Ordered: Blood cultures.
  Blood cultures positive for growth. Organism was identified.

Treatment Plan: Start patient on amphotericin B and IL-3 antitumor agent.

9/13/02: The patient returned with the usual signs of relapse. Continue chemotherapy and platelet transfusions as well as packed red blood cells. Follow up as outpatient.

LEARNING ACTIVITY

PATIENT: **Alfred Gates**

INSTRUCTIONS: *Before you begin, read the instructions carefully and follow each step in the process.*

STUDY GUIDES

Goal A

The goal in this activity is for you to relate laboratory data with Mr. Gates's symptoms on his admission to the hospital. This learning activity will allow you to collect and assess initial data pertaining to Mr. Gates.

Learning Issues

ISSUE 1: Identify physical findings presented by Mr. Gates that are considered typical for his diagnosed condition.

ISSUE 2: Determine the laboratory findings that are significant in the diagnosis of Mr. Gates's condition.

Study Questions A

1. Review the patient's medical records and determine which of the presenting symptoms and which elements of the background history the physician may consider significant in his illness.

CLINICAL SYMPTOMS:

BACKGROUND HISTORY:

_____

_____

_____

_____

2. In the space provided, list the laboratory tests that were requested at the time Mr. Gates was admitted to the facility. Which of the tests requested specifically correlate with his presenting symptoms? Highlight these tests.

_____

_____

_____

_____

3. Now access the laboratory test results from the Laboratory Information System (LIS) in the CD-ROM. Obtain Mr. Gates's results and record them on the patient laboratory test results forms provided in this workbook. Review Mr. Gates's laboratory test results at the time he was admitted to the hospital.

Note: If this is your first time accessing information in the CD-ROM, make sure that you start with "Before you begin."

4. a. Are any of the laboratory test results outside the usual acceptable range? If so, what do these results suggest?

_____

_____

_____

_____

b. What features observed on the peripheral blood and bone marrow smears are characteristic of Mr. Gates's diagnosed condition?

_____

_____

_____

5. Are there other laboratory findings that you consider significant in this case, given the background history of the patient (e.g., culture results)?

_____

_____

_____

_____

6. What diagnosis was made based on the clinical and laboratory findings?

_____

_____

_____

_____

7. Comment on the chemotherapeutic drug, cytarabine, that was prescribed for this patient. What precautions must patients observe while taking this drug, and what risks are they warned of?

_____

_____

_____

_____

Goal B

In this portion of the learning activity, the goal is for you to evaluate the patient's laboratory test results and determine how these results relate to his prognosis and ultimate outcome.

Learning Issues

ISSUE 1: Identify the consequences of organ transplantation and chemotherapy.

ISSUE 2: Consider the significance of the isolates recovered from organ transplant patients.

1. Access the **CD-ROM** for the identification of the organisms isolated from the sputum and blood cultures. Use the microbiology laboratory worksheets provided in this workbook to record the microscopic findings, biochemical tests performed, appropriate results, and identification of the organism(s). Evaluate the results. What organism(s) was (were) isolated from the blood cultures?

_____

_____

_____

_____

2. How do these findings correlate with Mr. Gates's clinical history?

_____

_____

_____

_____

3. What is the significance of this laboratory finding?

_____

_____

_____

_____

4. How is the classification (staging) system of Mr. Gates's condition defined? Based on his progress reports, what is the stage of his illness? What is the prognosis of his condition?

_____

_____

_____

_____

UNIVERSITY MEDICAL CENTER

Name: _____ Date: _____

Record #: _____ Time: _____

ANTIBODY IDENTIFICATION PANEL

Vial	Special Type	Donor	D	C	c	E	e	f	V	Cw	K	k	Kpa	Kpb	Jsa	Jsb	Fya	Fyb	Jka	Jkb	Lea	Leb	P1	M	N	S	s	LUa	LUb	Xga	#	37	AGH	CC
1	Bg(a+)	R1R1 B1080	+	+	0	0	+	0	0	0	0	+	0	+	0	+	+	0	0	+	0	+	+	+	+	+	+	0	+	+	1			
2		R1WR1 B1102	+	+	0	0	+	0	0	+	+	+	0	+	0	+	0	+	+	+	0	+	+	0	+	0	+	0	+	0	2			
3	Bg(a+)	R2R2 C1243	+	0	+	+	0	0	0	0	0	+	0	+	0	+	+	+	0	+	0	+	+	+	0	+	+	0	+	0	3			
4		ROR D575	+	0	+	0	+	+	0	0	0	+	0	+	0	+	0	0	+	0	+	0	+	+	+	0	+	0	+	+	4			
5		r'r E370	0	+	+	0	+	+	0	0	0	+	0	+	0	+	0	+	0	+	0	+	+	+	+	+	+	0	+	0	5			
6		r"r F416	0	0	+	+	0	+	0	0	0	+	0	+	0	+	+	0	+	+	+	0	0	+	0	0	+	+	+	+	6			
7		rrK G488	0	0	+	0	+	+	0	0	+	+	0	+	0	+	0	+	0	0	0	0	+	+	0	0	+	0	+	0	7			
8	Yt(b+)	rrFya H347	0	0	+	0	+	+	0	0	0	+	0	+	0	+	+	0	+	0	0	0	+	+	+	+	+	0	+	0	8			
9		rr N1434	0	0	+	0	+	+	0	0	0	+	0	+	0	+	+	+	+	+	+	0	+	+	+	+	0	0	+	+	9			
10	Co(b+)	R2R2 C199	+	0	+	+	0	0	0	0	0	+	0	+	0	+	+	+	0	0	0	0	0	+	0	0	+	0	+	+	10			
TC	He+	R1R2 A1086	+	+	+	+	+	0	0	0	0	+	0	+	0	+	0	0	+	+	0	+	+	+	+	0	+	+	+	0	TC			
		Patient's Cells																																

151

UNIVERSITY MEDICAL CENTER

Name: _____

Record #: _____

Date: _____

Time: _____

Cell Tests

Anti-A _____

Anti-B _____

Anti-D IS _____

Anti-D 37 _____

Anti-D AHG _____

Anti-A$_1$ Lectin _____

Serum Tests

	RT	37	AHG	CC
A$_1$ Cells	_____			
A$_2$ Cells	_____			
B Cells	_____			
Screen Cells I	_____	_____	_____	_____
Screen Cells II	_____	_____	_____	_____
Screen Cells III	_____	_____	_____	_____

UNIVERSITY MEDICAL CENTER
CONFIDENTIAL PATIENT INFORMATION
CUMULATIVE SUMMARY REPORT

PATIENT INFORMATION   ID number: _____   Ward: _____

Name: _____   Physician: _____

Address: _____   Date Admitted: _____

_____   Phone: _____

City: _____   State: _____   Zip: _____

Date of Birth: _____   Sex: _____   Race: _____

CHEMISTRY

Tests	Reference Ranges	Date: Time:	Date: Time:	Date: Time:	Date: Time:	Date: Time:
Acid Phos	2.5–11.7 U/L					
ACTH	9–52 pg/mL					
ALT	0–45 IU/L					
Albumin	3.5–5.0 g/dL					
A/G Ratio	0.7–2.1					
Aldosterone	??					
Alkaline Phos	41–137 IU/L					
Ammonia	11–35 µmol/L					
Amylase	95–290 U/L					
Anion Gap	10–18 mmol/L					
AST	0–41 IU/L					
Bilirubin	0.2–1.0 mg/dL					
Bilirubin (direct)	0.2–1.0 mg/dL					
BUN	10–20 mg/dL					
Calcium (total)	4.3–5.3 mEq/L					
Calcuim (ionized)	1.16–1.32 mmol/L					
Chloride	95–100 mmol/L					
Carbon Dioxide	23–32 mmol/L					

CHEMISTRY (page 2)

Tests	Reference Ranges	Date: Time:	Date: Time:	Date: Time:	Date: Time:	Date: Time:
Cholesterol	<200 mg/dL					
CK	15–160 U/L					
CK-MB	15–160 U/L					
Creatinine	0.7–1.5 mg/dL					
Creatintine Clearance	80–120 mL/min					
GGT	6–45 U/L					
Globulin	2.3–3.2 g/dL					
Glucose	65–105 mg/dL					
LD	100–225 U/L					
LDL Cholesterol	75–140 U/L					
LDL/HDL	2.9–2.2					
Lipase	0–1.0 U/mL					
Magnesium	1.3–2.1 mEq/L					
Osmolality	275–295 mOsM/kg					
Phosphorus	2.7–4.5 mg/dL					
Potassium	3.5–5.0 mmol/L					
Protein	5.8–8.2 g/dL					
Sodium	135–145 mmol/L					
Triglycerides	10–190 mg/dL					
Uric Acid	3.5–7.2 mg/dL					
HCO_3	100–225 U/L					

UNIVERSITY MEDICAL CENTER
CONFIDENTIAL PATIENT INFORMATION
CUMULATIVE SUMMARY REPORT

PATIENT INFORMATION   ID number: _____   Ward: _____

Name: _____   Physician: _____

Address: _____   Date Admitted: _____

_____   Phone: _____

City: _____   State: _____   Zip: _____

Date of Birth: _____   Sex: _____   Race: _____

HEMATOLOGY

Test	Reference Ranges	Date: Time:	Date: Time:	Date: Time:	Date: Time:	Date: Time:
Hemoglobin (g/dL) Male Female	14.0–18.0 12.0–15.0					
Hematocrit (%) Male Female	40–54 35–49					
RBC ($\times 10^{12}$/L) Male Female	4.6–6.6 4.0–5.4					
WBC ($\times 10^9$/L)	4.5–11.5					
MCV (fL)	80–94					
MCHC (g/dL or %)	32–36					
MCH (pg)	26–32					
Platelet Count ($\times 10^9$/L)	150–450					
RDW (%)	11.5–14.5					
Reticulocyte Count						
Segmented Neutrophils (%)	50–70					
Lymphocytes (%)	18–42					
Monocytes (%)	2–11					
Basophils (%)	0–2					
Eosinophils (%)	1–3					
Erythrocyte Sed Rate (ESR) Male Female	0–9 mm/hr 0–15 mm/hr					
Prothrombin Time (PT)	<2-sec deviation from control; 12–14 sec					
Activated Partial Thromboplastin Time (APTT)	<35 sec					
Fibrin Degradation Products (FDP)	4.9 ± 2.8 μg FDP/mL					
Thrombin Time	15 sec					
D-Dimer	<0.5 μg/mL					

UNIVERSITY MEDICAL CENTER

CONFIDENTIAL PATIENT INFORMATION
CUMULATIVE SUMMARY REPORT

PATIENT INFORMATION   ID number: _____   Ward: _____

Name: _____   Physician: _____

Address: _____   Date Admitted: _____

_____   Phone: _____

City: _____   State: _____   Zip: _____

Date of Birth: _____   Sex: _____   Race: _____

MICROBIOLOGY

Date and Time	Procedure / Specimen	Direct Smear	Preliminary Report	Final Report

CASE SUMMARY

A. Provide a brief summary of possible patient outcomes based on the laboratory test results and the patient's diagnoses.

_____

_____

_____

_____

_____

_____

_____

_____

B. Identify the learning points that you consider helpful in working up this patient's case. *(This will be an individual response.)*

_____

_____

_____

_____

_____

_____

_____

_____

_____

_____

NOTES

_____

_____

_____

_____

_____

_____

_____

_____

_____

▶ PATIENT'S RECORDS

PATIENT NAME: **Guya Ging**

PATIENT IDENTIFICATION NUMBER: **110548**

PHYSICIAN: **Dey**

PATIENT INFORMATION

NAME: Guya Ging   ID NUMBER: 110548

PHYSICIAN: Dey

DATE ADMITTED: 11/22/01   TIME: 300

ADDRESS: 826 Ino St., Sumware, SD 12345

PHONE: 200-222-5555

DATE OF BIRTH: 10/24/66 SEX: F   RACE: Asian   WARD: 2N

ADMISSION INFORMATION

WT.: 110 lb   HT.: 5'1"   B/P: 112/68

R: 24   PULSE: 88   TEMP.: 101.2

PRIMARY COMPLAINT

Fatigue, weakness, unexplained bruises

ADMISSION DIAGNOSIS

Thrombocytopenia

PATIENT HISTORY

This patient is a 35-year-old female who presented with complaints of fatigue for the past month. She also complained of easy bruising, especially on her arms and legs, and felt weak and feverish. She reported a 2-day history of bright red blood from her rectum. The patient also had a history of hypothyroidism. On physical examination, the patient showed pallor, was febrile, and appeared weak. The patient also revealed acute rectal bleeding, petechiae over her mouth, and ecchymoses on her arms and inner thighs.

TREATMENT PLAN

Laboratory Tests Ordered: CBC, coagulation studies, glucose, BUN, electrolytes, liver profile

Blood cultures ×2, type and cross-match for 2 units of packed red blood cells. Prepare 8 units of platelet concentrates for transfusion.

PROGRESS REPORTS

11/24/01, 1800: The patient received 8 units of platelets and 250 mL of packed red blood cells (RBCs). Blood culture preliminary reports are negative.

Treatment Plan: Evaluate coagulation, CBC, chemistry results. Request repeat of CBC. Request platelet counts and LDH daily.

11/25/01, 1000: The patient continued to show thrombocytopenia and intracellular hemolysis.

Treatment Plan: Request therapeutic plasma exchange (TPE).

Evaluate laboratory results. Continue the request for daily platelet counts. Monitor LDH values.

11/26/01, 0600: TPE was performed. Fresh frozen plasma was used as replacement fluid. The patient experienced perioral tingling and was treated to relieve the symptoms. She also had chills but no other problems during the therapeutic exchange procedure. The second procedure was planned for the next day.

11/29/01, 0900: The patient remained stable.

Treatment Plan: Transfuse packed RBCs as needed.

12/14/01, 0700: Twenty plasma exchanges of about 6 units of plasma per exchange were performed. Platelet count at 200,000/mL and LDH within reference range.

Patient was discharged from the hospital.

Treatment Plan: Schedule subsequent follow-up as outpatient visits.

PATIENT: **Guya Ging**

INSTRUCTIONS: *Before you begin, read the instructions carefully and follow each step in the process.*

STUDY GUIDES

Goal A

The goal in this activity is for you to relate laboratory data to Ms. Ging's medical history and clinical symptoms on her admission to the hospital. This learning activity will allow you to collect and assess initial data pertaining to Ms. Ging.

Learning Issues

ISSUE 1: Identify physical findings presented by Ms. Ging that are typical manifestations of her disease.

ISSUE 2: Determine how the differential diagnosis of this patient's condition was determined based on the clinical and laboratory findings.

Study Questions A

1. Review the patient's medical records and determine which of the presenting symptoms and which elements of the background history the physician may consider significant in her illness.

CLINICAL SYMPTOMS:

BACKGROUND HISTORY:

2. In the space provided, list the laboratory tests that were requested at the time of Ms. Ging's admission to the facility. Which of the tests requested specifically correlate with her presenting symptoms? Highlight these tests.

_____

_____

_____

_____

3. Now access the laboratory test results from the Laboratory Information System (LIS) in the CD-ROM. Obtain Ms. Ging's results and record them on the patient laboratory test results forms provided in this workbook. Review Ms. Ging's laboratory test results at the time she was admitted to the hospital.

4. a. Are any of the laboratory test results outside the usual acceptable range? If so, what do these results suggest?

_____

_____

_____

_____

b. How do these test results correlate with Ms. Ging's presenting symptoms?

_____

_____

_____

_____

5. Use the CD-ROM to review the peripheral blood smear. Observe the red blood cell morphology.

a. Comment on the red blood cell morphology.

_____

_____

_____

UNIVERSITY MEDICAL CENTER

Name: _____

Record #: _____

Date: _____

Time: _____

Cell Tests

Anti-A	_____
Anti-B	_____
Anti-D IS	_____
Anti-D 37	_____
Anti-D AHG	_____
Anti-A$_1$ Lectin	_____

Serum Tests

A$_1$ Cells	_____
A$_2$ Cells	_____
B Cells	_____

	RT	37	AHG	CC
Screen Cells I	___	___	___	___
Screen Cells II	___	___	___	___
Screen Cells III	___	___	___	___

167

UNIVERSITY MEDICAL CENTER
CONFIDENTIAL PATIENT INFORMATION
CUMULATIVE SUMMARY REPORT

PATIENT INFORMATION   ID number: _____   Ward: _____

Name: _____   Physician: _____

Address: _____   Date Admitted: _____

_____   Phone: _____

City: _____   State: _____   Zip: _____

Date of Birth: _____   Sex: _____   Race: _____

CHEMISTRY

Tests	Reference Ranges	Date: Time:	Date: Time:	Date: Time:	Date: Time:	Date: Time:
Acid Phos	2.5–11.7 U/L					
ACTH	9–52 pg/mL					
ALT	0–45 IU/L					
Albumin	3.5–5.0 g/dL					
A/G Ratio	0.7–2.1					
Aldosterone	??					
Alkaline Phos	41–137 IU/L					
Ammonia	11–35 µmol/L					
Amylase	95–290 U/L					
Anion Gap	10–18 mmol/L					
AST	0–41 IU/L					
Bilirubin	0.2–1.0 mg/dL					
Bilirubin (direct)	0.2–1.0 mg/dL					
BUN	10–20 mg/dL					
Calcium (total)	4.3–5.3 mEq/L					
Calcuim (ionized)	1.16–1.32 mmol/L					
Chloride	95–100 mmol/L					
Carbon Dioxide	23–32 mmol/L					

CHEMISTRY (page 2)

Tests	Reference Ranges	Date: Time:	Date: Time:	Date: Time:	Date: Time:	Date: Time:
Cholesterol	<200 mg/dL					
CK	15–160 U/L					
CK-MB	15–160 U/L					
Creatinine	0.7–1.5 mg/dL					
Creatintine Clearance	80–120 mL/min					
GGT	6–45 U/L					
Globulin	2.3–3.2 g/dL					
Glucose	65–105 mg/dL					
LD	100–225 U/L					
LDL Cholesterol	75–140 U/L					
LDL/HDL	2.9–2.2					
Lipase	0–1.0 U/mL					
Magnesium	1.3–2.1 mEq/L					
Osmolality	275–295 mOsM/kg					
Phosphorus	2.7–4.5 mg/dL					
Potassium	3.5–5.0 mmol/L					
Protein	5.8–8.2 g/dL					
Sodium	135–145 mmol/L					
Triglycerides	10–190 mg/dL					
Uric Acid	3.5–7.2 mg/dL					
HCO_3	100–225 U/L					

PATIENT INFORMATION   ID number: _____   Ward: _____

Name: _____   Physician: _____

Address: _____   Date Admitted: _____

_____   Phone: _____

City: _____   State: _____   Zip: _____

Date of Birth: _____   Sex: _____   Race: _____

HEMATOLOGY

Test	Reference Ranges	Date: Time:	Date: Time:	Date: Time:	Date: Time:	Date: Time:

Hemoglobin (g/dL)
  Male
  Female
	14.0–18.0
	12.0–15.0					

Hematocrit (%)
  Male
  Female
	40–54
	35–49					

RBC ($\times 10^{12}$/L)
  Male
  Female
	4.6–6.6
	4.0–5.4					

WBC ($\times 10^9$/L)	4.5–11.5					
MCV (fL)	80–94					
MCHC (g/dL or %)	32–36					
MCH (pg)	26–32					
Platelet Count ($\times 10^9$/L)	150–450					
RDW (%)	11.5–14.5					
Reticulocyte Count						
Segmented Neutrophils (%)	50–70					
Lymphocytes (%)	18–42					
Monocytes (%)	2–11					
Basophils (%)	0–2					
Eosinophils (%)	1–3					

Erythrocyte Sed Rate (ESR)
  Male
  Female
	0–9 mm/hr
	0–15 mm/hr					

Prothrombin Time (PT)	<2-sec deviation from control; 12–14 sec					
Activated Partial Thromboplastin Time (APTT)	<35 sec					
Fibrin Degradation Products (FDP)	4.9 ± 2.8 μg FDP/mL					
Thrombin Time	15 sec					
D-Dimer	<0.5 μg/mL					

UNIVERSITY MEDICAL CENTER
CONFIDENTIAL PATIENT INFORMATION
CUMULATIVE SUMMARY REPORT

PATIENT INFORMATION   ID number: _____   Ward: _____

Name: _____   Physician: _____

Address: _____   Date Admitted: _____

_____   Phone: _____

City: _____   State: _____   Zip: _____

Date of Birth: _____   Sex: _____   Race: _____

MICROBIOLOGY

Date and Time	Procedure / Specimen	Direct Smear	Preliminary Report	Final Report

CASE SUMMARY

A. Provide a brief summary of possible patient outcomes based on the laboratory test results and the patient's diagnoses.

_____

_____

_____

_____

_____

_____

_____

_____

B. Identify the learning points that you consider helpful in working up this patient's case. *(This will be an individual response.)*

_____

_____

_____

_____

_____

_____

_____

_____

_____

NOTES _____

_____

_____

_____

_____

_____

_____

_____

▶ PATIENT'S RECORDS

PATIENT NAME: **Janus Glass**

PATIENT IDENTIFICATION NUMBER: **135796**

PHYSICIAN: **Frazier**

PATIENT INFORMATION

NAME: Janus Glass   ID NUMBER: 135796

PHYSICIAN: Frazier

DATE ADMITTED: 03/18/01   TIME: 1100

ADDRESS: 257 Looney St., Sun City, NE 05678

PHONE: 210-666-4700

DATE OF BIRTH: 05/05/51   SEX: M   RACE: W   WARD: 3B

ADMISSION INFORMATION

WT.: 150 lb   HT.: 6'1"   B/P: 120/80

R: 24   PULSE: 110   TEMP.: 101

ADMISSION DIAGNOSIS

Pneumonia

PRIMARY COMPLAINT

Shortness of breath, hemoptysis, fatigue, weakness, productive cough

PATIENT HISTORY

This is a 49-year-old white male who was seen at the outpatient clinic for bacterial pneumonia follow-up. When seen at the clinic, the patient complained

173

of coughing up blood, very green sputum, weakness, fatigue, and shortness of breath. The patient was referred for inpatient admission. Physical findings on admission showed that the patient was febrile; chest x-ray showed chronic bullous lesions in the lungs, especially at the apical region. The patient denied night sweats or chills but had experienced slight weight loss with no apparent reason. His medical history included positive PPD and asbestos exposure. He revealed that he worked with insecticides on a farm. He reported heavy drinking and smoking three to four packages of tobacco products a week.

Treatment Plan

Radiology Ordered: Chest x-ray
Laboratory Tests Ordered: CBC, glucose, BUN, electrolytes, sputum direct smear, culture, PT, APTT

PROGRESS REPORTS

3/18/01, 1030: The patient developed a temperature spike of 101.7° F.

Treatment Plan:

Laboratory Tests Ordered: CBC, type and cross-match for 8 units of packed RBCs and fresh frozen plasma

3/18/01, 1300: Patient received 2 units of packed RBCs and 2 units of fresh frozen plasma.
Patient was scheduled for bronchoscopy.

3/19/01, 0800: Patient received 2 units of packed RBCs.

Treatment Plan: Bronchial washings for routine bacterial culture and acid-fast bacilli (AFB) and fungal cultures were requested.

3/22/01, 0800: The patient remained febrile with temperature spikes.
Patient received 2 units of packed RBCs.

Treatment Plan:

Laboratory Tests Ordered: CBC, hepatic enzymes, blood cultures
Bone marrow aspirates for AFB, fungal, and routine bacterial cultures.

3/25/01, 0800: Bone marrow aspirates showed intracellular yeasts. Patient was placed on amphotericin B. Patient received 2 units of packed RBCs.

Treatment Plan:

Laboratory Tests Ordered: WBC, hemoglobin/hematocrit, platelet count

3/31/01, 1000: Patient was not responding to amphotericin B.

Treatment Plan:

Laboratory Tests Ordered: WBC, hemoglobin/hematocrit, platelet count

4/07/01, 0800: Patient was deteriorating.

Treatment Plan:

Laboratory Tests Ordered: WBC, hemoglobin/hematocrit, platelet count, blood cultures, coagulation studies

Patient Progress: The patient did not respond to therapy. He expired 6 weeks from the day of admission.

LEARNING ACTIVITIES

PATIENT: **Janus Glass**

INSTRUCTIONS: *Before you begin, read the instructions carefully and follow each step in the process.*

STUDY GUIDES

Goal A

The goal in this activity is for you to determine how Mr. Glass's medical history and clinical symptoms may direct the clinician to a presumptive diagnosis.

Learning Issues

ISSUE 1: Identify factors in his medical and work history that predispose Mr. Glass to his condition.

ISSUE 2: Identify the significance of this information for your attempt to determine the etiologic agent of his infection.

Study Questions A

1. Review the patient's medical records and determine which of the presenting symptoms and which elements of the background history the physician may consider significant in his illness.

CLINICAL SYMPTOMS:

_____

_____

_____

_____

BACKGROUND HISTORY:

2. In the space provided, list the laboratory tests that were requested at the time of Mr. Glass's admission to the facility. Which of the tests requested specifically correlate with his presenting symptoms? Highlight these tests.

3. Now access the laboratory test results from the Laboratory Information System (LIS) in the CD-ROM. Obtain Mr. Glass's results and record them on the patient laboratory test results forms provided in this workbook. Review Mr. Glass's laboratory test results at the time he was admitted to the hospital.

   Note: If this is your first time accessing information in the CD-ROM, make sure that you start with "Before you begin."

4. a. Are any of the laboratory test results outside the usual acceptable range? If so, what do these results suggest?

   b. How do these test results correlate with Mr. Glass's presenting symptoms?

5. Are there other laboratory findings that you consider significant in this case, given the background history of the patient (e.g., culture results)?

6. What factors may have predisposed Mr. Glass to his current condition, based on his medical and work history?

7. What significance does this information have for your attempt to determine the etiologic agent of Mr. Glass's current infection?

Goal B

In this portion of the learning activity, the goal is for you to evaluate follow-up measures taken during the course of Mr. Glass's illness and how these measures relate to his prognosis and ultimate outcome.

Learning Issues

ISSUE 1: Identify the clinical manifestations Mr. Glass presents that direct the clinician to request bronchoscopy studies that include fungal and mycobacterial cultures and smears.

ISSUE 2: Determine why liver enzymes and blood culture studies are significant in monitoring this disease process.

UNIVERSITY MEDICAL CENTER
CONFIDENTIAL PATIENT INFORMATION
CUMULATIVE SUMMARY REPORT

PATIENT INFORMATION   ID number: _____   Ward: _____

Name: _____   Physician: _____

Address: _____   Date Admitted: _____

_____   Phone: _____

City: _____   State: _____   Zip: _____

Date of Birth: _____   Sex: _____   Race: _____

MICROBIOLOGY

Date and Time	Procedure / Specimen	Direct Smear	Preliminary Report	Final Report

CASE SUMMARY

A. Provide a brief summary of possible patient outcomes based on the laboratory test results and the patient's diagnoses.

_____

_____

_____

_____

_____

_____

_____

B. Identify the learning points that you consider helpful in working up this patient's case. *(This will be an individual response.)*

_____

_____

_____

_____

_____

_____

_____

NOTES

_____

_____

_____

_____

_____

_____

_____

_____

► PATIENT'S RECORDS

PATIENT NAME: **Roberto Guerero**

PATIENT IDENTIFICATION NUMBER: **323291**

PHYSICIAN: **Chilie**

PATIENT INFORMATION

NAME: Roberto Guerero   ID NUMBER: 323291

PHYSICIAN: Chilie

DATE ADMITTED: 03/21/01   TIME: 1300

ADDRESS: 625 Silver Grill Rd., Ridpath, WA 20037

PHONE: 000-502-4287

DATE OF BIRTH: 06/15/48   SEX: M   RACE: Hispanic

ADMISSION INFORMATION

WT.: 120 lb   HT.: 5'7"   B/P: 90/60

R: 18   PULSE: 76   TEMP.: 101

ADMISSION DIAGNOSIS
Staphylococcal or streptococcal cellulitis of the leg

PRIMARY COMPLAINT
Bilateral leg pains

PATIENT HISTORY
This is a 52-year-old Latin American male admitted through the ED with complaints of bilateral leg pains. The patient complained that the burning pain

was constant and started with his right lower calf. He reported that the pain increased in intensity and was accompanied by swelling within hours of onset. The patient also reported episodes of chills and fever. He denied vomiting or diarrhea.

Physical findings on admission showed that the patient was alert and oriented. His lungs were clear and his heart rate regular. His abdomen was soft and slightly protuberant, but there were no masses or enlargement of the spleen or liver. There was rash and tissue swelling on the left lower extremity. A surgical scar from a portacaval shunt put in place several years ago was evident.

The report of an endoscopic exam performed 15 days prior to admission showed duodenitis but no deformity, edema, or any evidence of ulcer.

The patient's previous history included Laënnec's cirrhosis, gastritis, and upper GI bleeding with several blood transfusions. A year previously, he was treated for cellulitis of the left leg. The patient had drunk three cases of beer per week for the past 10 years and smoked heavily.

TREATMENT PLAN

Oxacillin started.

Radiology Ordered: Chest x-ray

Laboratory Tests Ordered: Glucose, BUN, electrolytes, urinalysis, CBC, PT, APTT; culture of exudates from the leg; blood cultures

PROGRESS REPORTS

3/21/01, 1800: Patient was hypotensive, with rapid breathing and heart rate. Severely acidotic. The blisters had progressed from his lower extremities to his trunk and had developed into large bullae.

Treatment Plan: Antibiotic was changed to broad spectrum. Treatment for possible DIC and septic shock initiated.

3/22/01, 0600: Patient rapidly deteriorating. Patient went into DIC and septic shock. Unresponsive to therapy and attempts to improve blood pressure.

Treatment Plan: Place patient on mechanical ventilator.

3/22/01, 1700: Patient was unresponsive and expired.

LEARNING ACTIVITIES

PATIENT: Roberto Guerero

INSTRUCTIONS: *Before you begin, read the instructions carefully and follow each step in the process.*

STUDY GUIDES

Goal A

The goal in this activity is for you to relate laboratory findings with Mr. Guerero's previous medical history and his current clinical condition on admission to the hospital. This learning activity will allow you to collect and assess initial data pertaining to Mr. Guerero.

Learning Issues

ISSUE 1: Identify risk factors in his medical history that may have predisposed Mr. Guerero to his condition.

ISSUE 2: Identify possible causes of Mr. Guerero's condition, based on his presenting symptoms.

Study Questions A

1. Review the patient's medical records and determine which of the presenting symptoms and which elements of the background history the physician may consider significant in his illness.

CLINICAL SYMPTOMS:

_____

_____

_____

_____

BACKGROUND HISTORY:

_____

_____

_____

_____

2. In the space provided, list the laboratory tests that were requested at the time of Mr. Guerero's admission to the facility. Which of the tests requested specifically correlate with his presenting symptoms? Highlight these tests.

    _____

    _____

    _____

    _____

3. Now access the laboratory test results from the Laboratory Information System (LIS) in the CD-ROM. Obtain Mr. Guerero's results and record them on the patient laboratory test results forms provided in this workbook. Review Mr. Guerero's laboratory test results at the time he was admitted to the hospital.

    Note: If this is your first time accessing information in the CD-ROM, make sure that you start with "Before you begin."

4. Why is staphylococcal or streptococcal cellulitis suspected?

    _____

    _____

    _____

5. Are any of the laboratory test results outside the usual acceptable range? If so, what do these results suggest?

    _____

    _____

    _____

    _____

Goal B

In this portion of the learning activity, the goal is for you to evaluate follow-up test results on admission and how they relate to Mr. Guerero's clinical progress and ultimate outcome.

Learning Issues

ISSUE 1: Identify the laboratory tests that indicate the severity of Mr. Guerero's illness.

ISSUE 2: Evaluate the laboratory test results and identify findings that are significant in the patient's prognosis.

Study Questions B

1. Based on the PT and APTT results, what additional coagulation parameters are important in monitoring Mr. Guerero's progress? Use the CD-ROM to obtain the results of Mr. Guerero's additional laboratory tests. Record all laboratory findings on the patient laboratory tests results forms provided in this workbook.

2. What is the significance of these laboratory parameters?

3. What risk factors may have contributed to Mr. Guerero's fatal outcome?

4. Access the LIS on the CD-ROM for the identification of the organisms isolated from the exudate and blood cultures. Use the microbiology laboratory worksheets provided in this workbook to record the microscopic findings, biochemical tests performed, appropriate results, and identification of the organism(s). Evaluate the results. What organism(s) was (were) isolated from the exudate and blood cultures?

UNIVERSITY MEDICAL CENTER

Name: _____ Date: _____

Record #: _____ Time: _____

ANTIBODY IDENTIFICATION PANEL

Vial	Special Type	Donor	D	C	c	E	e	f	V	Cw	K	k	Kpa	Kpb	Jsa	Jsb	Fya	Fyb	Jka	Jkb	Lea	Leb	P1	M	N	S	s	LUa	LUb	Xga	37	AGH	CC	
							Rh-Hr						Kell				Duffy		Kidd		Lewis		P	MN				Lutheran		Xg	Test Methods			
1	Bg(a+)	R1R1 B1080	+	+	0	0	+	0	0	0	0	+	0	+	0	+	+	0	0	+	0	+	+	+	+	+	+	0	+	+				1
2		R1WR1 B1102	+	+	0	0	+	0	0	+	+	+	0	+	0	+	0	+	+	+	0	+	+	0	+	0	+	0	+	0				2
3	Bg(a+)	R2R2 C1243	+	0	+	+	0	0	0	0	0	+	0	+	0	+	+	+	0	+	0	+	+	+	0	+	+	0	+	+				3
4		ROR D575	+	0	+	0	+	+	0	0	0	+	0	+	0	+	0	+	+	0	0	0	+	0	+	0	+	0	+	+				4
5		r'r E370	0	+	+	0	+	+	0	0	0	+	0	+	0	+	+	+	0	+	0	+	+	+	+	+	+	0	+	0				5
6		r"r F416	0	0	+	+	+	+	0	0	0	+	0	+	0	+	0	+	+	+	+	0	0	+	+	0	+	+	+	+				6
7		rrK G488	0	0	+	0	+	+	0	0	+	+	0	+	0	+	0	0	0	+	0	0	0	+	0	0	+	0	+	0				7
8	Yt(b+)	rrFya H347	0	0	+	0	+	+	0	0	0	+	0	+	0	+	+	0	+	0	0	0	+	+	+	+	+	0	+	0				8
9		rr N1434	0	0	+	0	+	+	0	0	0	+	0	+	0	+	+	+	+	0	+	0	+	+	0	+	0	0	+	+				9
10	Co(b+)	R2R2 C199	+	0	+	+	0	0	0	0	0	+	0	+	0	+	+	+	+	0	+	0	+	+	+	0	+	0	+	+				10
TC	He+	R1R2 A1086	+	+	+	+	+	+	0	0	0	+	0	+	0	+	0	+	0	+	0	0	+	+	+	+	+	+	+	0				TC
		Patient's Cells																																

UNIVERSITY MEDICAL CENTER

Name: _____

Record #: _____

Date: _____

Time: _____

Cell Tests

Anti-A _____

Anti-B _____

Anti-D IS _____

Anti-D 37 _____

Anti-D AHG _____

Anti-A_1 Lectin _____

Serum Tests

	RT	37	AHG	CC
A_1 Cells	_____			
A_2 Cells	_____			
B Cells	_____			
Screen Cells I	_____	_____	_____	_____
Screen Cells II	_____	_____	_____	_____
Screen Cells III	_____	_____	_____	_____

UNIVERSITY MEDICAL CENTER
CONFIDENTIAL PATIENT INFORMATION
CUMULATIVE SUMMARY REPORT

PATIENT INFORMATION

ID number: _____ Ward: _____

Name: _____ Physician: _____

Address: _____ Date Admitted: _____

_____ Phone: _____

City: _____ State: _____ Zip: _____

Date of Birth: _____ Sex: _____ Race: _____

CHEMISTRY

Tests	Reference Ranges	Date: Time:	Date: Time:	Date: Time:	Date: Time:	Date: Time:
Acid Phos	2.5–11.7 U/L					
ACTH	9–52 pg/mL					
ALT	0–45 IU/L					
Albumin	3.5–5.0 g/dL					
A/G Ratio	0.7–2.1					
Aldosterone	??					
Alkaline Phos	41–137 IU/L					
Ammonia	11–35 µmol/L					
Amylase	95–290 U/L					
Anion Gap	10–18 mmol/L					
AST	0–41 IU/L					
Bilirubin	0.2–1.0 mg/dL					
Bilirubin (direct)	0.2–1.0 mg/dL					
BUN	10–20 mg/dL					
Calcium (total)	4.3–5.3 mEq/L					
Calcuim (ionized)	1.16–1.32 mmol/L					
Chloride	95–100 mmol/L					
Carbon Dioxide	23–32 mmol/L					

CHEMISTRY (page 2)

Tests	Reference Ranges	Date: Time:	Date: Time:	Date: Time:	Date: Time:	Date: Time:
Cholesterol	<200 mg/dL					
CK	15–160 U/L					
CK-MB	15–160 U/L					
Creatinine	0.7–1.5 mg/dL					
Creatintine Clearance	80–120 mL/min					
GGT	6–45 U/L					
Globulin	2.3–3.2 g/dL					
Glucose	65–105 mg/dL					
LD	100–225 U/L					
LDL Cholesterol	75–140 U/L					
LDL/HDL	2.9–2.2					
Lipase	0–1.0 U/mL					
Magnesium	1.3–2.1 mEq/L					
Osmolality	275–295 mOsM/kg					
Phosphorus	2.7–4.5 mg/dL					
Potassium	3.5–5.0 mmol/L					
Protein	5.8–8.2 g/dL					
Sodium	135–145 mmol/L					
Triglycerides	10–190 mg/dL					
Uric Acid	3.5–7.2 mg/dL					
HCO_3	100–225 U/L					

PATIENT INFORMATION   ID number: _____   Ward: _____

Name: _____   Physician: _____

Address: _____   Date Admitted: _____

_____   Phone: _____

City: _____   State: _____   Zip: _____

Date of Birth: _____   Sex: _____   Race: _____

HEMATOLOGY

Test	Reference Ranges	Date: Time:	Date: Time:	Date: Time:	Date: Time:	Date: Time:
Hemoglobin (g/dL) Male Female	14.0–18.0 12.0–15.0					
Hematocrit (%) Male Female	40–54 35–49					
RBC ($\times 10^{12}$/L) Male Female	4.6–6.6 4.0–5.4					
WBC ($\times 10^{9}$/L)	4.5–11.5					
MCV (fL)	80–94					
MCHC (g/dL or %)	32–36					
MCH (pg)	26–32					
Platelet Count ($\times 10^{9}$/L)	150–450					
RDW (%)	11.5–14.5					
Reticulocyte Count						
Segmented Neutrophils (%)	50–70					
Lymphocytes (%)	18–42					
Monocytes (%)	2–11					
Basophils (%)	0–2					
Eosinophils (%)	1–3					
Erythrocyte Sed Rate (ESR) Male Female	0–9 mm/hr 0–15 mm/hr					
Prothrombin Time (PT)	<2-sec deviation from control; 12–14 sec					
Activated Partial Thromboplastin Time (APTT)	<35 sec					
Fibrin Degradation Products (FDP)	4.9 ± 2.8 µg FDP/mL					
Thrombin Time	15 sec					
D-Dimer	<0.5 µg/mL					

UNIVERSITY MEDICAL CENTER
CONFIDENTIAL PATIENT INFORMATION
CUMULATIVE SUMMARY REPORT

PATIENT INFORMATION   ID number: _____   Ward: _____

Name: _____   Physician: _____

Address: _____   Date Admitted: _____

_____   Phone: _____

City: _____   State: _____   Zip: _____

Date of Birth: _____   Sex: _____   Race: _____

MICROBIOLOGY

Date and Time	Procedure / Specimen	Direct Smear	Preliminary Report	Final Report

CASE SUMMARY

A. Provide a brief summary of possible patient outcomes based on the laboratory test results and the patient's diagnoses.

_____

_____

_____

_____

_____

_____

_____

B. Identify the learning points that you consider helpful in working up this patient's case. *(This will be an individual response.)*

_____

_____

_____

_____

_____

_____

_____

_____

NOTES

_____

_____

_____

_____

_____

_____

_____

▶ PATIENT'S RECORDS

PATIENT NAME: **Mei Lin**

PATIENT IDENTIFICATION NUMBER: **562341**

PHYSICIAN: **Edison**

PATIENT INFORMATION

NAME: Mei Lin   ID NUMBER: 562341

PHYSICIAN: Edison

DATE ADMITTED: 7/12/02   TIME: 1840

ADDRESS: 2110 N. Eye, Crossroad, MD 22220

PHONE: 000-555-3355

DATE OF BIRTH: 6/27/79   SEX: F   RACE: Asian

ADMISSION INFORMATION

WT.: 140 lb   HT.: 5'1"   B/P: 120/74

R: 17   PULSE: 83   TEMP.: 97.3

MEDICATION:

ADMISSION DIAGNOSIS
Pregnant, in labor at full term

PRIMARY COMPLAINT
Abdominal contractions

PATIENT HISTORY

The patient, a 23-year-old Asian female, moved to the area 1 month ago. This is the first time she is being seen at this hospital. There are no prenatal care records available at the time of admission. All prenatal care was provided at another hospital. The last visit to the previous hospital was 3 months ago. The patient had no complications during this pregnancy and is at full term, ready for delivery of the child. The patient has had one previous pregnancy and delivery of a healthy child 3 years ago at the previous hospital. The patient has never been transfused and is not taking any prescription medications.

TREATMENT PLAN

Laboratory Tests Ordered: CBC, urinalysis, electrolytes, glucose, BUN

PROGRESS REPORTS

6/12/03, 0200: The patient delivered a 7-lb baby boy with no complications.

Treatment Plan: Following delivery, evaluate the patient for Rh immune globulin (RhIG) eligibility and evaluate the child for potential hemolytic disease of the newborn (HDN) risk.

Request copies of prenatal work-up from the other hospital where the patient had previously been seen.

6/13/03, 1800: Review laboratory test results.

Treatment Plan: Administer RhIG. Discharge patient. Provide patient with information on well-baby clinic follow-up visits.

LEARNING ACTIVITIES

PATIENT: Mei Lin

INSTRUCTIONS: *Before you begin, read the instructions carefully and follow each step in the process.*

STUDY GUIDES

Goal A

The goal in this activity is for you to relate laboratory data with Ms. Lin's symptoms on her admission to the hospital. This learning activity will allow you to collect and assess initial data pertaining to Ms. Lin.

Learning Issues

ISSUE 1: From the clinician's notes, identify relevant signs and symptoms, social and previous medical history, and results of the physical examination.

ISSUE 2: Identify significant laboratory findings that are related to Ms. Lin's clinical condition. Review the laboratory test results provided in the documentation and determine the rationale for the clinician's course of action.

Study Questions A

1. Review the patient's medical records and determine which of the presenting symptoms and which elements of the background history the physician may consider significant in her illness.

CLINICAL SYMPTOMS:

_____

_____

_____

_____

BACKGROUND HISTORY:

_____

_____

_____

_____

2. In the space provided, list the laboratory tests requested at the time of Ms. Lin's admission. Which of the tests requested specifically correlate with her presenting symptoms? Highlight these tests.

_____

_____

_____

_____

3. Now access the laboratory test results from the Laboratory Information System (LIS) in the CD-ROM. Obtain Ms. Lin's results on admission and record them on the patient laboratory tests results forms provided in this workbook. Review Ms. Lin's laboratory test results at the time she was admitted to the hospital.

    Note: If this is your first time accessing information in the CD-ROM, make sure that you start with "Before you begin."

4. a. Are any of the laboratory test results outside the usual acceptable range? List those results that are outside the usual acceptable range.

    _____

    _____

    _____

    _____

    b. What do these results indicate?

    _____

    _____

    _____

    _____

Goal B

In this portion of the learning activity, the goal is for you to evaluate follow-up measures taken regarding Ms. Lin's condition. This learning activity will allow you to identify discrepancies in laboratory test results and understand how these issues are resolved with additional testing if needed.

Learning Issues

ISSUE 1: Interpret the data obtained and provide the appropriate product(s) for this patient.

ISSUE 2: Evaluate the use of the laboratory in this case.

1. Access the laboratory test results from the LIS in the CD-ROM. Obtain Ms. Lin's laboratory test results after she delivered her baby and record them on the patient laboratory test results forms provided in this workbook. Review the test results and the interpretation of those results provided.

2. a. What is the ABO/Rh group of the patient? Is the patient a candidate for RhIG?

    b. Review the remaining test results (antibody screen, antibody iden-tification, and test for fetomaternal hemorrhage).

3. a. What tests need to be performed in order to determine the RhIG eligibility for the patient and the HDN risk for the child?

    b. Is the child at risk for HDN? Support your answer.

4. How would you determine the origin of the anti-D in the patient?

5. Review the patient's records from the other hospital. Is the patient a candidate for RhIG? Support your answer.

6. a. How do you determine the quantity of RhIG to administer to the patient? What quantity of RhIG should be administered to this patient?

   b. What is the risk of the patient's producing immune-stimulated anti-D following this second dose of RhIG?

   c. What would be the risk if the patient did not receive the initial dose of RhIG at 28 weeks' gestation?

   d. What would be the risk if the patient did not receive any doses of RhIG during this pregnancy?

UNIVERSITY MEDICAL CENTER

Name: _____   Date: _____

Record #: _____   Time: _____

ANTIBODY IDENTIFICATION PANEL

Special Type	Vial	Donor	D	C	c	E	e	f	V	Cw	K	k	Kpa	Kpb	Jsa	Jsb	Fya	Fyb	Jka	Jkb	Lea	Leb	P1	M	N	S	s	LUa	LUb	Xga	#	37	AGH	CC
																												Lua	Lub	Xga		37	AGH	CC
			D	C	c	E	e	f	V	Cw	K	k	Kpa	Kpb	Jsa	Jsb	Fya	Fyb	Jka	Jkb	Lea	Leb	P1	M	N	S	s							
Bg(a+)	1	R1R1 B1080	+	+	0	0	+	0	0	0	0	+	0	+	0	+	+	0	0	+	0	+	+	+	+	+	+	0	+	+	1			
	2	R1WR1 B1102	+	+	0	0	+	0	0	+	+	+	0	+	0	+	0	+	+	+	0	+	+	0	+	0	+	0	+	0	2			
Bg(a+)	3	R2R2 C1243	+	0	+	+	0	0	0	0	0	+	0	+	0	+	+	0	0	+	0	+	+	+	0	+	0	0	+	+	3			
	4	ROR D575	+	0	+	0	+	+	0	0	0	+	0	+	0	+	0	0	+	0	0	0	+	0	+	0	+	0	+	+	4			
	5	r'r E370	0	+	+	0	+	+	0	0	0	+	0	+	0	+	+	+	0	+	0	+	+	+	+	+	+	0	+	0	5			
	6	r"r F416	0	0	+	+	+	+	0	0	0	+	0	+	0	+	0	+	+	+	0	+	0	+	+	0	+	+	+	+	6			
	7	rrK G488	0	0	+	0	+	+	0	0	+	+	0	+	0	+	0	+	0	+	+	0	0	+	0	0	+	0	+	0	7			
Yt(b+)	8	rrFya H347	0	0	+	0	+	+	0	0	0	+	0	+	0	+	+	0	+	0	+	0	+	+	+	+	+	0	+	0	8			
	9	rr N1434	0	0	+	0	+	+	0	0	0	+	0	+	0	+	+	+	+	+	0	+	+	+	+	0	0	0	+	+	9			
Co(b+)	10	R2R2 C199	+	0	+	+	0	0	0	0	0	+	0	+	0	+	+	0	+	0	+	0	0	+	+	0	+	0	+	+	10			
He+	TC	R1R2 A1086	+	+	+	+	+	+	0	0	0	+	0	+	0	+	0	+	+	0	0	+	+	+	+	+	+	+	+	0	TC			
		Patient's Cells																																

UNIVERSITY MEDICAL CENTER

Name: _____

Date: _____

Record #: _____

Time: _____

Cell Tests

Anti-A _____

Anti-B _____

Anti-D IS _____

Anti-D 37 _____

Anti-D AHG _____

Anti-A$_1$ Lectin _____

Serum Tests

A$_1$ Cells _____

A$_2$ Cells _____

B Cells _____

	RT	37	AHG	CC
Screen Cells I	___	___	___	___
Screen Cells II	___	___	___	___
Screen Cells III	___	___	___	___

UNIVERSITY MEDICAL CENTER
CONFIDENTIAL PATIENT INFORMATION
CUMULATIVE SUMMARY REPORT

PATIENT INFORMATION   ID number: _____   Ward: _____

Name: _____   Physician: _____

Address: _____   Date Admitted: _____

_____   Phone: _____

City: _____   State: _____   Zip: _____

Date of Birth: _____   Sex: _____   Race: _____

CHEMISTRY

Tests	Reference Ranges	Date: Time:	Date: Time:	Date: Time:	Date: Time:	Date: Time:
Acid Phos	2.5–11.7 U/L					
ACTH	9–52 pg/mL					
ALT	0–45 IU/L					
Albumin	3.5–5.0 g/dL					
A/G Ratio	0.7–2.1					
Aldosterone	??					
Alkaline Phos	41–137 IU/L					
Ammonia	11–35 μmol/L					
Amylase	95–290 U/L					
Anion Gap	10–18 mmol/L					
AST	0–41 IU/L					
Bilirubin	0.2–1.0 mg/dL					
Bilirubin (direct)	0.2–1.0 mg/dL					
BUN	10–20 mg/dL					
Calcium (total)	4.3–5.3 mEq/L					
Calcuim (ionized)	1.16–1.32 mmol/L					
Chloride	95–100 mmol/L					
Carbon Dioxide	23–32 mmol/L					

CHEMISTRY (page 2)

Tests	Reference Ranges	Date: Time:	Date: Time:	Date: Time:	Date: Time:	Date: Time:
Cholesterol	<200 mg/dL					
CK	15–160 U/L					
CK-MB	15–160 U/L					
Creatinine	0.7–1.5 mg/dL					
Creatintine Clearance	80–120 mL/min					
GGT	6–45 U/L					
Globulin	2.3–3.2 g/dL					
Glucose	65–105 mg/dL					
LD	100–225 U/L					
LDL Cholesterol	75–140 U/L					
LDL/HDL	2.9–2.2					
Lipase	0–1.0 U/mL					
Magnesium	1.3–2.1 mEq/L					
Osmolality	275–295 mOsM/kg					
Phosphorus	2.7–4.5 mg/dL					
Potassium	3.5–5.0 mmol/L					
Protein	5.8–8.2 g/dL					
Sodium	135–145 mmol/L					
Triglycerides	10–190 mg/dL					
Uric Acid	3.5–7.2 mg/dL					
HCO_3	100–225 U/L					

UNIVERSITY MEDICAL CENTER
CONFIDENTIAL PATIENT INFORMATION
CUMULATIVE SUMMARY REPORT

PATIENT INFORMATION   ID number: _____   Ward: _____

Name: _____   Physician: _____

Address: _____   Date Admitted: _____

_____   Phone: _____

City: _____   State: _____   Zip: _____

Date of Birth: _____   Sex: _____   Race: _____

HEMATOLOGY

Test	Reference Ranges	Date: Time:	Date: Time:	Date: Time:	Date: Time:	Date: Time:
Hemoglobin (g/dL) Male Female	14.0–18.0 12.0–15.0					
Hematocrit (%) Male Female	40–54 35–49					
RBC ($\times 10^{12}$/L) Male Female	4.6–6.6 4.0–5.4					
WBC ($\times 10^9$/L)	4.5–11.5					
MCV (fL)	80–94					
MCHC (g/dL or %)	32–36					
MCH (pg)	26–32					
Platelet Count ($\times 10^9$/L)	150–450					
RDW (%)	11.5–14.5					
Reticulocyte Count						
Segmented Neutrophils (%)	50–70					
Lymphocytes (%)	18–42					
Monocytes (%)	2–11					
Basophils (%)	0–2					
Eosinophils (%)	1–3					
Erythrocyte Sed Rate (ESR) Male Female	0–9 mm/hr 0–15 mm/hr					
Prothrombin Time (PT)	<2-sec deviation from control; 12–14 sec					
Activated Partial Thromboplastin Time (APTT)	<35 sec					
Fibrin Degradation Products (FDP)	4.9 ± 2.8 µg FDP/mL					
Thrombin Time	15 sec					
D-Dimer	<0.5 µg/mL					

UNIVERSITY MEDICAL CENTER
CONFIDENTIAL PATIENT INFORMATION
CUMULATIVE SUMMARY REPORT

PATIENT INFORMATION   ID number: _____   Ward: _____

Name: _____   Physician: _____

Address: _____   Date Admitted: _____

_____   Phone: _____

City: _____   State: _____   Zip: _____

Date of Birth: _____   Sex: _____   Race: _____

MICROBIOLOGY

Date and Time	Procedure / Specimen	Direct Smear	Preliminary Report	Final Report

CASE SUMMARY

A. Provide a brief summary of possible patient outcomes based on the laboratory test results and the patient's diagnoses.

_____

_____

_____

_____

_____

_____

_____

_____

B. Identify the learning points that you consider helpful in working up this patient's case. *(This will be an individual response.)*

_____

_____

_____

_____

_____

_____

_____

_____

NOTES

_____

_____

_____

_____

_____

▶ PATIENT'S RECORDS

PATIENT NAME: **Minh Sang Ngo**

PATIENT IDENTIFICATION NUMBER: **182008**

PHYSICIAN: **Mikey**

PATIENT INFORMATION

NAME: Minh Sang Ngo   ID NUMBER: 182008

PHYSICIAN: Mikey

DATE ADMITTED: 2/04/02   TIME: 300

ADDRESS: 1320 New Haven, San Antonio, TX 78235

PHONE: 210-656-5555

DATE OF BIRTH: 1/28/95   SEX: M   RACE: Asian   WARD: 2S

ADMISSION INFORMATION

WT.: 100 lb   HT.: 4'5"   B/P: 102/71

R: 15   PULSE: 76   TEMP.: 101.2

PRIMARY COMPLAINT

Fever, fatigue, anorexia, unexplained bruises

ADMISSION DIAGNOSIS

Thrombocytopenia

PATIENT HISTORY

The patient is a 7-year-old male child who presented with an epithelial disorder 5 days after a bone marrow transplant. Six months prior, the child was seen at the clinic for fatigue, pallor, and fever of unknown cause. The child tired easily and showed bruising on his extremities. Evaluation of laboratory test results provided the diagnosis. In spite of an aggressive chemotherapy, the child showed signs of relapse; hence, an autologous bone marrow transplant was performed. On this admission, physical examination showed that the child was febrile and showed a papule with a necrotic center on the right calf and a new lesion on the left finger.

TREATMENT PLAN

Laboratory Tests Ordered: Blood culture × 3; bacterial, fungal, and AFB cultures of biopsied lesion; CBC, coagulation studies, glucose, BUN, electrolytes

PROGRESS REPORTS

2/06/02, 1800: The patient received 6 units of platelets and 250 mL of packed RBCs. Blood culture results pending. AFB smear on tissue biopsy showed "no AFB seen." Fungal and bacterial direct smears showed "no organisms seen."

Treatment Plan: Evaluate CBC, chemistry results. Request bone marrow aspiration. Review immunologic cell surface markers.

2/07/02, 1000: The patient remained stable. AFB and fungal cultures of tissue still pending.

Treatment Plan: Evaluate preliminary blood culture results.

2/08/02, 0600: The patient remained stable. Evaluated blood culture results and culture results of lesions.

2/11/02, 0900: Evaluated bone marrow aspiration results and cell surface markers.

2/13/02, 0700: Suspected graft-versus-host disease (GVHD).

Treatment Plan: Discharge patient from the hospital. Discuss with patient's parents chemotherapy and supportive transfusions as options.

LEARNING ACTIVITIES

PATIENT: Minh Sang Ngo

INSTRUCTIONS: *Before you begin, read the instructions carefully and follow each step in the process.*

STUDY GUIDES

Goal A

The goal in this activity is for you to relate laboratory findings with Mr. Ngo's symptoms on his admission to the hospital. This learning activity will allow you to collect and assess initial data pertaining to Mr. Ngo.

Learning Issues

ISSUE 1: Identify physical findings presented by Mr. Ngo that are considered typical for his diagnosed condition.

ISSUE 2: Identify the laboratory findings that correlate with the clinical signs and symptoms.

ISSUE 3: Determine the significance of immunologic cell markers in the diagnosis of Mr. Ngo's disease.

Study Questions A

1. Review the patient's medical records and determine which of the presenting symptoms and which elements of the background history the physician may consider significant in his illness.

CLINICAL SYMPTOMS:

_____

_____

_____

_____

BACKGROUND HISTORY:

_____

_____

_____

_____

2. In the space provided, list the laboratory tests that were requested at the time of Mr. Ngo's admission to the facility. Which of the tests requested specifically correlate with his presenting symptoms? Highlight these tests.

_____

_____

_____

_____

3. Now access the laboratory test results from the Laboratory Information System (LIS) in the CD-ROM. Obtain Mr. Ngo's results and record them on the patient laboratory tests results forms provided in this workbook.

     Note: If this is your first time accessing information in the CD-ROM, make sure that you start with "Before you begin."

4. Are any of the laboratory results outside the usual acceptable range? If so, list the tests that are outside the acceptable range.

_____

_____

_____

_____

5. How do these test results correlate with Mr. Ngo's presenting symptoms, and what do these results suggest?

_____

_____

_____

_____

6. a. What diagnosis was made based on the cell morphology seen on the peripheral blood smear and bone marrow aspirates?

_____

_____

_____

b. What criteria were used in the diagnosis of this patient's illness?

c. What additional procedures were performed to confirm the diagnosis? Why are these procedures important?

7. Compare the chromosomal analysis performed most recently with an earlier analysis result. Explain your observations.

Goal B

In this portion of the learning activity, the goal is for you to evaluate the patient's laboratory test results and determine how these results relate to his diagnosis, prognosis, and ultimate outcome.

Learning Issues

ISSUE 1: Consider the significance of the request to perform blood cultures and tissue biopsy studies.

ISSUE 2: Evaluate the use of the laboratory in this case.

Study Questions B

1. a. Based on the patient's progress reports, chemotherapy failed and the patient showed signs of relapse. What options are available to this patient?

    _____

    _____

    _____

    _____

    b. What consequences may occur if these options fail?

    _____

    _____

    _____

    _____

2. a. Access the CD-ROM for the identification of the organisms isolated from the tissue and blood cultures. Use the microbiology laboratory worksheets provided in this workbook to record the microscopic findings, biochemical tests performed, appropriate results, and identification of the organism(s). Evaluate the results. What organism(s) was (were) isolated from the blood and tissue cultures?

    _____

    _____

    _____

    _____

    b. Do you agree with the results? Why or why not? *(This will be an individual response.)*

    _____

    _____

    _____

    _____

   c. What is the significance of these results?

_____

_____

_____

_____

3. a. What is GVHD?

_____

_____

_____

_____

   b. Why does GVHD occur?

_____

_____

_____

_____

   c. What are the signs and symptoms of GVHD?

_____

_____

_____

_____

   d. Are there ways to prevent or minimize the risk for GVHD?

_____

_____

_____

_____

UNIVERSITY MEDICAL CENTER

Name: _____ Date: _____

Record #: _____ Time: _____

ANTIBODY IDENTIFICATION PANEL

Vial	Special Type	Donor	D	C	c	E	e	f	V	Cw	K	k	Kpa	Kpb	Jsa	Jsb	Fya	Fyb	JKa	JKb	Lea	Leb	P1	M	N	S	s	LUa	LUb	Xga	37	AGH	CC	
1	Bg(a+)	R1R1 B1080	+	+	0	0	+	0	0	0	0	+	0	+	0	+	+	0	0	+	0	+	+	+	+	+	+	0	+	+				1
2		R1WR1 B1102	+	+	0	0	+	0	0	+	+	+	0	+	0	+	0	+	+	+	0	+	+	0	+	0	+	0	+	0				2
3	Bg(a+)	R2R2 C1243	+	0	+	+	0	0	0	0	0	+	0	+	0	+	0	+	0	+	0	+	+	+	0	+	+	0	+	+				3
4		ROR D575	+	0	+	0	+	+	0	0	0	+	0	+	0	+	0	0	+	0	0	0	+	+	+	0	+	0	+	+				4
5		r'r E370	0	+	+	0	+	+	0	0	0	+	0	+	0	+	+	0	0	+	0	+	+	+	+	+	+	+	+	0				5
6		r"r F416	0	0	+	+	+	+	0	0	0	+	0	+	0	+	0	+	+	+	0	+	0	+	0	0	+	+	+	+				6
7		rrK G488	0	0	+	0	+	+	0	0	+	+	0	+	0	+	0	+	0	+	+	0	0	+	0	0	+	0	+	0				7
8	Yt(b+)	rrFya H347	0	0	+	0	+	+	0	0	0	+	0	+	0	+	+	0	+	0	+	0	+	+	+	+	+	0	+	0				8
9		rrN1434	0	0	+	0	+	+	0	0	0	+	0	+	0	+	+	+	+	+	0	+	0	+	0	+	0	0	+	+				9
10	Co(b+)	R2R2 C199	+	0	+	+	0	0	0	0	0	+	0	+	0	+	+	+	+	0	0	+	+	+	+	0	+	0	+	+				10
TC	He+	R1R2 A1086	+	+	+	+	+	0	0	0	0	+	0	+	0	+	0	+	0	+	0	+	+	+	+	+	+	+	+	0				TC
		Patient's Cells																																

UNIVERSITY MEDICAL CENTER

Name: _____

Record #: _____

Date: _____

Time: _____

Cell Tests

Anti-A _____

Anti-B _____

Anti-D IS _____

Anti-D 37 _____

Anti-D AHG _____

Anti-A_1 Lectin _____

Serum Tests

	RT	37	AHG	CC
A_1 Cells	_____			
A_2 Cells	_____			
B Cells	_____			
Screen Cells I	_____	_____	_____	_____
Screen Cells II	_____	_____	_____	_____
Screen Cells III	_____	_____	_____	_____

UNIVERSITY MEDICAL CENTER
CONFIDENTIAL PATIENT INFORMATION
CUMULATIVE SUMMARY REPORT

PATIENT INFORMATION   ID number: _____   Ward: _____

Name: _____   Physician: _____

Address: _____   Date Admitted: _____

_____   Phone: _____

City: _____   State: _____   Zip: _____

Date of Birth: _____   Sex: _____   Race: _____

CHEMISTRY

Tests	Reference Ranges	Date: Time:	Date: Time:	Date: Time:	Date: Time:	Date: Time:
Acid Phos	2.5–11.7 U/L					
ACTH	9–52 pg/mL					
ALT	0–45 IU/L					
Albumin	3.5–5.0 g/dL					
A/G Ratio	0.7–2.1					
Aldosterone	??					
Alkaline Phos	41–137 IU/L					
Ammonia	11–35 μmol/L					
Amylase	95–290 U/L					
Anion Gap	10–18 mmol/L					
AST	0–41 IU/L					
Bilirubin	0.2–1.0 mg/dL					
Bilirubin (direct)	0.2–1.0 mg/dL					
BUN	10–20 mg/dL					
Calcium (total)	4.3–5.3 mEq/L					
Calcuim (ionized)	1.16–1.32 mmol/L					
Chloride	95–100 mmol/L					
Carbon Dioxide	23–32 mmol/L					

CHEMISTRY (page 2)

Tests	Reference Ranges	Date: Time:	Date: Time:	Date: Time:	Date: Time:	Date: Time:
Cholesterol	<200					
CK	15–160 U/L					
CK-MB	15–160 U/L					
Creatinine	0.7–1.5 mg/dL					
Creatintine Clearance	80–120 mL/min					
GGT	6–45 U/L					
Globulin	2.3–3.2 g/dL					
Glucose	65–105 mg/dL					
LD	100–225 U/L					
LDL Cholesterol	75–140 U/L					
LDL/HDL	2.9–2.2					
Lipase	0–1.0 U/mL					
Magnesium	1.3–2.1 mEq/L					
Osmolality	275–295mOsM/kg					
Phosphorus	2.7–4.5 mg/dL					
Potassium	3.5–5.0 mmol/L					
Protein	5.8–8.2 g/dL					
Sodium	135–145 mmol/L					
Triglycerides	10–190 mg/dL					
Uric Acid	3.5–7.2 mg/dL					
HCO_3	100–225 U/L					

PATIENT INFORMATION ID number: _____ Ward: _____

Name: _____ Physician: _____

Address: _____ Date Admitted: _____

_____ Phone: _____

City: _____ State: _____ Zip: _____

Date of Birth: _____ Sex: _____ Race: _____

HEMATOLOGY

Test	Reference Ranges	Date: Time:	Date: Time:	Date: Time:	Date: Time:	Date: Time:
Hemoglobin (g/dL) Male Female	14.0–18.0 12.0–15.0					
Hematocrit (%) Male Female	40–54 35–49					
RBC ($\times 10^{12}$/L) Male Female	4.6–6.6 4.0–5.4					
WBC ($\times 10^{9}$/L)	4.5–11.5					
MCV (fL)	80–94					
MCHC (g/dL or %)	32–36					
MCH (pg)	26–32					
Platelet Count ($\times 10^{9}$/L)	150–450					
RDW (%)	11.5–14.5					
Reticulocyte Count						
Segmented Neutrophils (%)	50–70					
Lymphocytes (%)	18–42					
Monocytes (%)	2–11					
Basophils (%)	0–2					
Eosinophils (%)	1–3					
Erythrocyte Sed Rate (ESR) Male Female	0–9 mm/hr 0–15 mm/hr					
Prothrombin Time (PT)	<2-sec deviation from control; 12–14 sec					
Activated Partial Thromboplastin Time (APTT)	<35 sec					
Fibrin Degradation Products (FDP)	4.9 ± 2.8 µg FDP/mL					
Thrombin Time	15 sec					
D-Dimer	<0.5 µg/mL					

UNIVERSITY MEDICAL CENTER
CONFIDENTIAL PATIENT INFORMATION
CUMULATIVE SUMMARY REPORT

PATIENT INFORMATION   ID number: _____   Ward: _____

Name: _____   Physician: _____

Address: _____   Date Admitted: _____

_____   Phone: _____

City: _____   State: _____   Zip: _____

Date of Birth: _____   Sex: _____   Race: _____

MICROBIOLOGY

Date and Time	Procedure / Specimen	Direct Smear	Preliminary Report	Final Report

CASE SUMMARY

A. Provide a brief summary of possible patient outcomes based on the laboratory test results and the patient's diagnoses.

B. Identify the learning points that you consider helpful in working up this patient's case. *(This will be an individual response.)*

NOTES

► PATIENT'S RECORDS

PATIENT NAME: **George Pitt**

PATIENT IDENTIFICATION NUMBER: **581450**

PHYSICIAN: **McCarthy**

PATIENT INFORMATION

NAME: George Pitt   ID NUMBER: 581450

PHYSICIAN: McCarthy

DATE ADMITTED: 6/03/98   TIME: 0600

ADDRESS: 8723 No. Bend, Landing, VA 22222

PHONE: 000-555-5544

DATE OF BIRTH: 2/5/67   SEX: M   RACE: B

ADMISSION INFORMATION

WT.: 120   HT.: 5'10"   B/P: 150/90

R: 17   PULSE: 83   TEMP.: 102.3

MEDICATION:

ADMISSION DIAGNOSIS

Acute appendicitis

PRIMARY COMPLAINT

Pain on his right side, nausea, fever

PATIENT HISTORY

The patient is a 31-year-old African American male who has had an unexplained dull pain in his right side, vomiting, and diarrhea for the last 3 days. This morning he felt nauseous and feverish and had a sharp pain in the same area. The patient was seen at this hospital 3 years ago. At that time, he had ingested a toothpick that damaged his digestive tract to the point where surgery was required to remove the toothpick and repair the injuries. Because of a low hemoglobin/hematocrit following the surgery, the patient was transfused 2 units of red blood cells. The patient has not been seen at any other hospital. He is not taking any medications.

TREATMENT PLAN

Laboratory Tests Ordered: CBC, electrolytes, PT, APTT

Physician Orders: Emergency surgery to remove the patient's appendix. Two units of red blood cells if needed during or following surgery.

PROGRESS REPORTS

6/3/98, 1100: Following the procedure, the patient's hematocrit has fallen and he is having difficulty breathing.

Treatment Plan: Transfuse 2 units of red blood cell products.

6/5/98, 1000: The patient was stable and was discharged from the hospital. Postsurgical follow-up in outpatient clinic in 7 days.

6/8/98, Outpatient Visit: Three days postdischarge, the patient returned to the hospital with complaints of weakness and fever.

Treatment Plan: Readmit patient.

Laboratory Tests Ordered: CBC, bilirubin, blood cultures × 3

6/8/98, Readmission: Examined for and showed no signs of any postsurgical bleed. Reviewed blood culture reports. Investigate for a transfusion reaction.

Treatment Plan: Transfusion reaction investigation.

6/9/98: The patient appeared stable and afebrile.

Treatment Plan: Patient to be discharged on 6/10 if temperature remains normal. Repeat hemoglobin and hematocrit on 6/10. Follow up in physician's office in 3 days.

PATIENT: George Pitt

INSTRUCTIONS: *Before you begin, read the instructions carefully and follow each step in the process.*

STUDY GUIDES

Goal A

The goal in this activity is for you to relate laboratory data with Mr. Pitt's symptoms on his admission to the hospital. This learning activity will allow you to collect and assess initial data pertaining to Mr. Pitt.

Learning Issues

ISSUE 1: From the clinician's notes, identify relevant signs and symptoms, social and previous medical history, and results of the physical examination.

ISSUE 2: Identify significant laboratory findings that are related to Mr. Pitt's clinical condition at the time of presentation. Correlate these findings with his clinical presentation.

ISSUE 3: Review the laboratory test results provided in the documentation and identify discrepancies, if any, that may need to be resolved.

Study Questions A

1. Review the patient's medical records and determine which of the presenting symptoms and which elements of the background history the physician may consider significant in his illness.

CLINICAL SYMPTOMS:

BACKGROUND HISTORY:

_____

_____

_____

_____

2. In the space provided, list the laboratory tests that were requested at the time of Mr. Pitt's admission. Which of the tests requested specifically correlate with his presenting symptoms? Highlight these tests.

_____

_____

_____

_____

3. Now access the laboratory test results from the Laboratory Information System (LIS) in the CD-ROM. Obtain Mr. Pitt's laboratory test results on admission and record them on the patient laboratory tests results forms provided in this workbook. Review Mr. Pitt's laboratory test results at the time he was admitted to the hospital.
    Note: If this is your first time accessing information in the CD-ROM, make sure that you start with "Before you begin."

4. a. Are any of the laboratory test results outside the usual acceptable range? List those results that are outside the usual acceptable range.

_____

_____

_____

_____

    b. What do these results indicate?

_____

_____

_____

_____

5. Following the procedure, the patient's hematocrit had fallen and the patient complained of having difficulty breathing. The physician requested that the patient receive 2 units of red blood cell products. Access the blood bank transfusion records from the LIS in the CD-ROM. Obtain Mr. Pitt's compatibility test results and record them on the forms provided in this workbook. Based on the compatibility test results, would you issue the products?

_____

_____

_____

_____

Goal B

In this portion of the learning activity, the goal is for you to evaluate follow-up measures taken regarding Mr. Pitt's condition. This learning activity will allow you to identify discrepancies in laboratory test results and understand how these issues are resolved with additional testing if needed.

Learning Issues

ISSUE 1: Interpret the data obtained and provide the appropriate blood product(s) for this patient.

ISSUE 2: Evaluate the use of the laboratory in this case.

Study Questions B

1. Three days following the surgery, the patient returned to the hospital. Access Mr. Pitt's laboratory test results from the LIS in the CD-ROM. Obtain Mr. Pitt's laboratory results on his second admission and record them on the patient laboratory tests results forms provided in this workbook. Review the test results and the interpretation of those results that is provided.

2. a. Given the laboratory test results, what could be some causes of the patient's condition?

_____

_____

_____

_____

b. Which of the laboratory tests requested may confirm the suspected cause of the patient's current condition?

_____

_____

_____

_____

3. a. What items are to be sent to the blood bank laboratory for a transfusion reaction investigation?

_____

_____

_____

b. What tests must be performed by the blood bank laboratory as part of an initial transfusion reaction investigation?

_____

_____

_____

_____

4. Review the initial transfusion reaction investigation results. Based on these results, how would you proceed in your investigation? List the additional tests that must be performed. Review the test results obtained by the blood bank. Why is it important to perform these procedures?

_____

_____

_____

5. The physician wants to rule out a laboratory testing error as a cause of this transfusion reaction.

a. What tests can be performed to rule out a laboratory testing error in this case?

_____

_____

_____

_____

b. Review the blood bank records and test findings. How would you categorize this transfusion reaction? How is it different from other types of transfusion reactions?

_____

_____

_____

_____

c. What could have been done to prevent this transfusion reaction from occurring in this patient?

_____

_____

_____

d. What can be done to prevent this transfusion reaction from occurring again in this patient?

_____

_____

_____

_____

CASE SUMMARY

UNIVERSITY MEDICAL CENTER

Name: _____ Date: _____

Record #: _____ Time: _____

ANTIBODY IDENTIFICATION PANEL

Vial	Special Type	Donor	Rh-Hr								Kell						Duffy		Kidd		Lewis		P	MN				Lutheran		Xg	Test Methods		
			D	C	c	E	e	f	V	Cw	K	k	Kpa	Kpb	Jsa	Jsb	Fya	Fyb	Jka	Jkb	Lea	Leb	P1	M	N	S	s	LUa	LUb	Xga	37	AGH	CC
1	Bg(a+)	R1R1 B1080	+	+	0	0	+	0	0	0	0	+	0	+	0	+	+	0	0	+	0	+	+	+	+	+	+	0	+	+			1
2		R1WR1 B1102	+	+	0	0	+	0	0	+	+	+	0	+	0	+	0	+	+	+	0	+	+	0	+	0	+	0	+	0			2
3	Bg(a+)	R2R2 C1243	+	0	+	+	0	0	0	0	0	+	0	+	0	+	+	+	0	+	0	+	+	+	0	+	+	0	+	+			3
4		ROR D575	+	0	+	0	+	+	0	0	0	+	0	+	0	+	0	0	+	0	0	0	+	+	+	0	+	0	+	+			4
5		r'r E370	0	+	+	0	+	+	0	0	0	+	0	+	0	+	+	+	0	+	0	+	+	+	+	+	+	0	+	0			5
6		r"r F416	0	0	+	+	+	+	0	0	0	+	0	+	0	+	0	+	+	+	0	+	+	+	+	0	+	+	+	+			6
7		rrK G488	0	0	+	0	+	+	0	0	+	+	0	+	0	+	0	+	+	0	+	0	0	+	0	0	+	0	+	0			7
8	Yt(b+)	rrFya H347	0	0	+	0	+	+	0	0	0	+	0	+	0	+	+	+	+	+	+	0	+	+	+	+	0	0	+	0			8
9		rr N1434	0	0	+	0	+	+	0	0	0	+	0	+	0	+	+	+	+	0	0	+	0	+	0	0	+	0	+	+			9
10	Co(b+)	R2R2 C199	+	0	+	+	0	0	0	0	0	+	0	+	0	+	+	+	+	0	+	0	0	+	+	0	+	0	+	+			10
TC	He+	R1R2 A1086	+	+	+	+	+	0	0	0	0	+	0	+	0	+	0	0	0	+	0	+	+	+	+	+	+	+	+	0			TC
		Patient's Cells																															

Name: _____

Record #: _____

Date: _____

Time: _____

Cell Tests

Anti-A _____

Anti-B _____

Anti-D IS _____

Anti-D 37 _____

Anti-D AHG _____

Anti-A$_1$ Lectin _____

Serum Tests

	RT	37	AHG	CC
A$_1$ Cells	_____			
A$_2$ Cells	_____			
B Cells	_____			
Screen Cells I	_____	_____	_____	_____
Screen Cells II	_____	_____	_____	_____
Screen Cells III	_____	_____	_____	_____

235

UNIVERSITY MEDICAL CENTER
CONFIDENTIAL PATIENT INFORMATION
CUMULATIVE SUMMARY REPORT

PATIENT INFORMATION   ID number: _____   Ward: _____

Name: _____   Physician: _____

Address: _____   Date Admitted: _____

_____   Phone: _____

City: _____   State: _____   Zip: _____

Date of Birth: _____   Sex: _____   Race: _____

CHEMISTRY

Tests	Reference Ranges	Date: Time:	Date: Time:	Date: Time:	Date: Time:	Date: Time:
Acid Phos	2.5–11.7 U/L					
ACTH	9–52 pg/mL					
ALT	0–45 IU/L					
Albumin	3.5–5.0 g/dL					
A/G Ratio	0.7–2.1					
Aldosterone	??					
Alkaline Phos	41–137 IU/L					
Ammonia	11–35 μmol/L					
Amylase	95–290 U/L					
Anion Gap	10–18 mmol/L					
AST	0–41 IU/L					
Bilirubin	0.2–1.0 mg/dL					
Bilirubin (direct)	0.2–1.0 mg/dL					
BUN	10–20 mg/dL					
Calcium (total)	4.3–5.3 mEq/L					
Calcuim (ionized)	1.16–1.32 mmol/L					
Chloride	95–100 mmol/L					
Carbon Dioxide	23–32 mmol/L					

CHEMISTRY (page 2)

Tests	Reference Ranges	Date: Time:	Date: Time:	Date: Time:	Date: Time:	Date: Time:
Cholesterol	<200 mg/dL					
CK	15–160 U/L					
CK-MB	15–160 U/L					
Creatinine	0.7–1.5 mg/dL					
Creatintine Clearance	80–120 mL/min					
GGT	6–45 U/L					
Globulin	2.3–3.2 g/dL					
Glucose	65–105 mg/dL					
LD	100–225 U/L					
LDL Cholesterol	75–140 U/L					
LDL/HDL	2.9–2.2					
Lipase	0–1.0 U/mL					
Magnesium	1.3–2.1 mEq/L					
Osmolality	275–295 mOsM/kg					
Phosphorus	2.7–4.5 mg/dL					
Potassium	3.5–5.0 mmol/L					
Protein	5.8–8.2 g/dL					
Sodium	135–145 mmol/L					
Triglycerides	10–190 mg/dL					
Uric Acid	3.5–7.2 mg/dL					
HCO_3	100–225 U/L					

CONFIDENTIAL PATIENT INFORMATION
CUMULATIVE SUMMARY REPORT

PATIENT INFORMATION   ID number: _____   Ward: _____

Name: _____   Physician: _____

Address: _____   Date Admitted: _____

_____   Phone: _____

City: _____   State: _____   Zip: _____

Date of Birth: _____   Sex: _____   Race: _____

HEMATOLOGY

Test	Reference Ranges	Date: Time:	Date: Time:	Date: Time:	Date: Time:	Date: Time:
Hemoglobin (g/dL)						
Male	14.0–18.0					
Female	12.0–15.0					
Hematocrit (%)						
Male	40–54					
Female	35–49					
RBC ($\times 10^{12}$/L)						
Male	4.6–6.6					
Female	4.0–5.4					
WBC ($\times 10^{9}$/L)	4.5–11.5					
MCV (fL)	80–94					
MCHC (g/dL or %)	32–36					
MCH (pg)	26–32					
Platelet Count ($\times 10^{9}$/L)	150–450					
RDW (%)	11.5–14.5					
Reticulocyte Count						
Segmented Neutrophils (%)	50–70					
Lymphocytes (%)	18–42					
Monocytes (%)	2–11					
Basophils (%)	0–2					
Eosinophils (%)	1–3					
Erythrocyte Sed Rate (ESR)						
Male	0–9 mm/hr					
Female	0–15 mm/hr					
Prothrombin Time (PT)	<2-sec deviation from control; 12–14 sec					
Activated Partial Thromboplastin Time (APTT)	<35 sec					
Fibrin Degradation Products (FDP)	4.9 ± 2.8 µg FDP/mL					
Thrombin Time	15 sec					
D-Dimer	<0.5 µg/mL					

UNIVERSITY MEDICAL CENTER
CONFIDENTIAL PATIENT INFORMATION
CUMULATIVE SUMMARY REPORT

PATIENT INFORMATION   ID number: _____   Ward: _____

Name: _____   Physician: _____

Address: _____   Date Admitted: _____

_____   Phone: _____

City: _____   State: _____   Zip: _____

Date of Birth: _____   Sex: _____   Race: _____

MICROBIOLOGY

Date and Time	Procedure / Specimen	Direct Smear	Preliminary Report	Final Report

A. Provide a brief summary of possible patient outcomes based on the laboratory test results and the patient's diagnoses.

_____

_____

_____

_____

_____

_____

_____

B. Identify the learning points that you consider helpful in working up this patient's case. *(This will be an individual response.)*

_____

_____

_____

_____

_____

_____

_____

_____

_____

NOTES

_____

_____

_____

_____

_____

_____

_____

_____

► PATIENT'S RECORDS

PATIENT NAME: **Walter Reeve**

PATIENT IDENTIFICATION NUMBER: **681460**

PHYSICIAN: **McArthur**

PATIENT INFORMATION

NAME: Walter Reeve   ID NUMBER: 681460

PHYSICIAN: McArthur

DATE ADMITTED: 8/30/88   TIME: 0840

ADDRESS: 1230 So. Bench, Ware, VA 22222

PHONE: 000-555-5544

DATE OF BIRTH: 5/5/73   SEX: M   RACE: W

ADMISSION INFORMATION

WT.: 132 lb   HT.: 5'10"   B/P: 158/94

R: 17   PULSE: 83   TEMP.: 97.3

MEDICATION:

ADMISSION DIAGNOSIS
Rule out fractured hip

PRIMARY COMPLAINT
Dizziness, bruises on the hip, weak

PATIENT HISTORY

The patient, a 15-year-old male Caucasian, was transported to the hospital by his parent after falling off a dining room chair. The patient was standing on the chair changing a ceiling light bulb when he lost his balance and fell to the floor. The patient landed on his hip, but was able to quickly stand and walk off the injury. One hour later, the patient felt light-headed and weak. The patient and the patient's parent observed a 6-in-diameter, dark purple bruise on the patient's hip. The patient was born at the hospital without complications, and his medical history revealed no visits to any medical facilities other than for routine checkups. The patient has never been transfused and is taking no medications. An interview with the parent and the patient revealed a history of small hematomas following minor bumps on the knee. No professional medical care was obtained to treat these 1-in-diameter bruises. The bruises disappeared on their own. The patient was admitted for observation.

TREATMENT PLAN

Radiology Ordered: X-ray of hip area
Laboratory Tests Ordered: Hemoglobin, hematocrit, bleeding time, PT, APTT

PROGRESS REPORTS

8/30/88, 1000: Reviewed laboratory results. X-ray of hip area showed no broken bones.

Treatment Plan: Request factor assay. Proceed with treatment plan.

LEARNING ACTIVITIES

PATIENT: Walter Reeve
INSTRUCTIONS: *Before you begin, read the instructions carefully and follow each step in the process.*

STUDY GUIDES

Goal A

The goal in this activity is for you to relate laboratory data with Mr. Reeve's symptoms on his admission to the hospital. This learning activity will allow you to collect and assess initial data pertaining to Mr. Reeve.

Learning Issues

ISSUE 1: From the clinician's notes, identify relevant signs and symptoms, social and previous medical history, and results of the physical examination.

ISSUE 2: Identify significant laboratory findings that are related to Mr. Reeve's clinical condition at the time of presentation. Correlate these findings with his clinical presentation.

ISSUE 3: Review the laboratory test results provided in the documentation and identify discrepancies, if any, that may need to be resolved.

Study Questions A

1. Review the patient's medical records and determine which of the presenting symptoms and which elements of the background history the physician may consider significant in his illness.

CLINICAL SYMPTOMS:

_____

_____

_____

_____

BACKGROUND HISTORY:

_____

_____

_____

_____

2. In the space provided, list the laboratory tests that were requested at the time of Mr. Reeve's admission. Which of the tests requested specifically correlate with his presenting symptoms? Highlight these tests.

_____

_____

_____

_____

3. Now access the laboratory test results from the Laboratory Information System (LIS) in the CD-ROM. Obtain Mr. Reeve's laboratory results on admission and record them on the patient laboratory tests results forms provided in this workbook. Review Mr. Reeve's laboratory test results at the time he was admitted to the hospital.

   Note: If this is your first time accessing information in the CD-ROM, make sure that you start with "Before you begin."

4. a. Are any of the laboratory test results outside the usual acceptable range? List those results that are outside the usual acceptable range.

_____

_____

_____

_____

   b. What do these results indicate?

_____

_____

_____

_____

Goal B

In this portion of the learning activity, the goal is for you to evaluate follow-up measures taken regarding Mr. Reeve's condition. This learning activity will allow you to identify discrepancies in laboratory test results and understand how these issues are resolved with additional testing if needed.

Learning Issues

ISSUE 1: Interpret the data obtained and provide the appropriate blood product(s) for this patient.

ISSUE 2: Evaluate the use of the laboratory in this case.

Study Questions B

1. Review the laboratory test results that you obtained from the LIS in Learning Activity A3. Review the test results and the interpretation of the results provided.

2. Given the initial laboratory test results, what additional tests should be run to complete the diagnosis?

_____

_____

_____

_____

3. What information does the additional testing provide for this case?

_____

_____

_____

_____

4. If the physician wants to treat the patient by raising his factor VIII level to 0.50 unit/mL, what is the best product to administer to the patient?

_____

_____

_____

_____

5. What amount of factor VIII should be administered to the patient in order to raise his factor VIII to the requested level?

_____

_____

_____

_____

6. If the physician wants to use cryoprecipitate to treat the patient, how many bags of product should be administered?

_____

_____

_____

_____

7. The patient has a previous ABO/Rh type of A positive on file in the blood bank records. Is a new specimen required for testing prior to the administration of either of these products? Provide your rationale for your answer.

_____

_____

_____

_____

8. What should be the ABO/Rh type of the cryoprecipitate products that are prepared for the patient?

    _____

    _____

    _____

    _____

9. If the factor VIII level of a pool of 14 bags of cryoprecipitate is found to be 1200 units, is this an acceptable product?

    _____

    _____

    _____

    _____

10. Is the laboratory appropriately used for this patient? Explain. *(This will be an individual response.)*

    _____

    _____

    _____

Name: _____   Date: _____

Record #: _____   Time: _____

ANTIBODY IDENTIFICATION PANEL

Vial	Special Type	Donor	Rh-Hr D	C	c	E	e	f	V	Cw	Kell K	k	Kpa	Kpb	Jsa	Jsb	Duffy Fya	Fyb	Kidd Jka	Jkb	Lewis Lea	Leb	P P1	MN M	N	S	s	Lutheran LUa	LUb	Xg Xga	#	Test Methods 37	AGH	CC
1	Bg(a+)	R1R1 B1080	+	+	0	0	+	0	0	0	0	+	0	+	0	+	+	0	0	+	0	+	+	+	+	+	+	0	+	+	1			
2		R1WR1 B1102	+	+	0	0	+	0	0	+	+	+	0	+	0	+	0	+	+	+	0	+	+	0	+	0	+	0	+	0	2			
3	Bg(a+)	R2R2 C1243	+	0	+	+	0	0	0	0	0	+	0	+	0	+	+	+	0	+	0	+	+	+	0	+	+	0	+	+	3			
4		ROR D575	+	0	+	0	+	+	0	0	0	+	0	+	0	+	0	0	+	0	0	0	+	0	+	0	+	0	+	+	4			
5		r'r E370	0	+	+	0	+	+	0	0	0	+	0	+	0	+	+	+	0	+	0	+	+	+	+	0	+	0	+	0	5			
6		r"r F416	0	0	+	+	+	+	0	0	0	+	0	+	0	+	0	+	+	+	0	+	0	+	+	0	+	+	+	+	6			
7		rrK G488	0	0	+	0	+	+	0	0	+	+	0	+	0	+	+	+	+	+	+	0	0	+	0	0	+	0	+	0	7			
8	Yt(b+)	rrFya H347	0	0	+	0	+	+	0	0	0	+	0	+	0	+	0	0	+	0	+	0	+	+	+	+	+	0	+	0	8			
9		rr N1434	0	0	+	0	+	+	0	0	0	+	0	+	0	+	+	+	+	+	0	+	+	+	0	+	0	0	+	+	9			
10	Co(b+)	R2R2 C199	+	0	+	+	0	0	0	0	0	+	0	+	0	+	+	+	+	0	+	0	+	+	+	0	+	0	+	+	10			
TC	He+	R1R2 A1086	+	+	+	+	+	0	0	0	0	+	0	+	0	+	0	0	0	+	0	+	+	+	+	+	+	+	+	0	TC			
		Patient's Cells																																

UNIVERSITY MEDICAL CENTER

Name: _____   Date: _____

Record #: _____   Time: _____

Cell Tests

Anti-A _____

Anti-B _____

Anti-D IS _____

Anti-D 37 _____

Anti-D AHG _____

Anti-A_1 Lectin _____

Serum Tests

A_1 Cells _____

A_2 Cells _____

B Cells _____

	RT	37	AHG	CC
Screen Cells I	___	___	___	___
Screen Cells II	___	___	___	___
Screen Cells III	___	___	___	___

UNIVERSITY MEDICAL CENTER
CONFIDENTIAL PATIENT INFORMATION
CUMULATIVE SUMMARY REPORT

PATIENT INFORMATION   ID number: _____   Ward: _____

Name: _____   Physician: _____

Address: _____   Date Admitted: _____

_____   Phone: _____

City: _____   State: _____   Zip: _____

Date of Birth: _____   Sex: _____   Race: _____

CHEMISTRY

Tests	Reference Ranges	Date: Time:	Date: Time:	Date: Time:	Date: Time:	Date: Time:
Acid Phos	2.5–11.7 U/L					
ACTH	9–52 pg/mL					
ALT	0–45 IU/L					
Albumin	3.5–5.0 g/dL					
A/G Ratio	0.7–2.1					
Aldosterone	??					
Alkaline Phos	41–137 IU/L					
Ammonia	11–35 μmol/L					
Amylase	95–290 U/L					
Anion Gap	10–18 mmol/L					
AST	0–41 IU/L					
Bilirubin	0.2–1.0 mg/dL					
Bilirubin (direct)	0.2–1.0 mg/dL					
BUN	10–20 mg/dL					
Calcium (total)	4.3–5.3 mEq/L					
Calcuim (ionized)	1.16–1.32 mmol/L					
Chloride	95–100 mmol/L					
Carbon Dioxide	23–32 mmol/L					

CHEMISTRY (page 2)

Tests	Reference Ranges	Date: Time:	Date: Time:	Date: Time:	Date: Time:	Date: Time:
Cholesterol	<200 mg/dL					
CK	15–160 U/L					
CK-MB	15–160 U/L					
Creatinine	0.7–1.5 mg/dL					
Creatintine Clearance	80–120 mL/min					
GGT	6–45 U/L					
Globulin	2.3–3.2 g/dL					
Glucose	65–105 mg/dL					
LD	100–225 U/L					
LDL Cholesterol	75–140 U/L					
LDL/HDL	2.9–2.2					
Lipase	0–1.0 U/mL					
Magnesium	1.3–2.1 mEq/L					
Osmolality	275–295 mOsM/kg					
Phosphorus	2.7–4.5 mg/dL					
Potassium	3.5–5.0 mmol/L					
Protein	5.8–8.2 g/dL					
Sodium	135–145 mmol/L					
Triglycerides	10–190 mg/dL					
Uric Acid	3.5–7.2 mg/dL					
HCO_3	100–225 U/L					

PATIENT INFORMATION   ID number: _____   Ward: _____

Name: _____   Physician: _____

Address: _____   Date Admitted: _____

_____   Phone: _____

City: _____   State: _____   Zip: _____

Date of Birth: _____   Sex: _____   Race: _____

HEMATOLOGY

Test	Reference Ranges	Date: Time:	Date: Time:	Date: Time:	Date: Time:	Date: Time:
Hemoglobin (g/dL) 　Male 　Female	 14.0–18.0 12.0–15.0					
Hematocrit (%) 　Male 　Female	 40–54 35–49					
RBC ($\times 10^{12}$/L) 　Male 　Female	 4.6–6.6 4.0–5.4					
WBC ($\times 10^{9}$/L)	4.5–11.5					
MCV (fL)	80–94					
MCHC (g/dL or %)	32–36					
MCH (pg)	26–32					
Platelet Count ($\times 10^{9}$/L)	150–450					
RDW (%)	11.5–14.5					
Reticulocyte Count						
Segmented Neutrophils (%)	50–70					
Lymphocytes (%)	18–42					
Monocytes (%)	2–11					
Basophils (%)	0–2					
Eosinophils (%)	1–3					
Erythrocyte Sed Rate (ESR) 　Male 　Female	 0–9 mm/hr 0–15 mm/hr					
Prothrombin Time (PT)	<2-sec deviation from control; 12–14 sec					
Activated Partial Thromboplastin Time (APTT)	<35 sec					
Fibrin Degradation Products (FDP)	4.9 ± 2.8 µg FDP/mL					
Thrombin Time	15 sec					
D-Dimer	<0.5 µg/mL					

UNIVERSITY MEDICAL CENTER
CONFIDENTIAL PATIENT INFORMATION
CUMULATIVE SUMMARY REPORT

PATIENT INFORMATION   ID number: _____   Ward: _____

Name: _____   Physician: _____

Address: _____   Date Admitted: _____

_____   Phone: _____

City: _____   State: _____   Zip: _____

Date of Birth: _____   Sex: _____   Race: _____

MICROBIOLOGY

Date and Time	Procedure / Specimen	Direct Smear	Preliminary Report	Final Report

CASE SUMMARY

A. Provide a brief summary of possible patient outcomes based on the laboratory test results and the patient's diagnoses.

_____
_____
_____
_____
_____
_____
_____

B. Identify the learning points that you consider helpful in working up this patient's case. *(This will be an individual response.)*

_____
_____
_____
_____
_____
_____
_____
_____
_____

NOTES

_____
_____
_____
_____
_____
_____
_____
_____

► PATIENT'S RECORDS

PATIENT NAME: **Paul L. Richmond**

PATIENT IDENTIFICATION NUMBER: **971250**

PHYSICIAN: **Lennon**

PATIENT INFORMATION

NAME: Paul L. Richmond   ID NUMBER: 971250

PHYSICIAN: Lennon

DATE ADMITTED: 6/30/01   TIME: 0840

ADDRESS: 5355 Guthrie, East Point, GA 00550

PHONE: 000-555-4589

DATE OF BIRTH: 6/14/38   SEX: M   RACE: W

ADMISSION INFORMATION

WT.: 232 lb   HT.: 6'2"   B/P: 154/90

R: 17   PULSE: 90   TEMP.: 97.3

MEDICATION: Mevacor daily

ADMISSION DIAGNOSIS
Chest pain; rule out AMI

PRIMARY COMPLAINT
Chest tightness

PATIENT HISTORY

The patient is a 63-year-old white male who presented to the ED with a 2-day history of chest tightness and discomfort. On the morning of 6/28 he mowed his lawn with a riding lawnmower, and 15 min after finishing he began to have pain between his shoulder blades and into his back. It lasted approximately 90 min and spontaneously resolved. Later that afternoon he worked in the yard again, and the same sort of discomfort occurred. This episode lasted about an hour before resolving. On 6/29, he attempted to complete his yard work and experienced another period of pain that lasted approximately an hour. Mild nausea, but no vomiting or shortness of breath, occurred during these episodes. He contacted his primary physician and was advised to go to the ED but decided against that advice, since he was feeling better. On 6/30 he had a recurrence of the pain without exertion and came to the hospital for evaluation.

The patient has long-standing hyperlipidemia that has not been controlled well with diet and medication and a history of percutaneous transluminal coronary angioplasty 8 years previously. No cardiac problems have been noted since the procedure. Patient history is positive for cigarette smoking (1 pack/day for 25 years) and negative for drug or alcohol use.

FAMILY HISTORY

Mother and father died of heart attacks, and a brother is currently being treated for coronary artery disease.

Patient was admitted to CCU for monitoring of cardiac function.

TREATMENT PLAN

Laboratory Tests Ordered: CBC, UA, CMP, cardiac profile, ABG, lipid profile
Other Tests Ordered: ECG

Antianginal medications and analgesics administered as needed.

PROGRESS REPORTS

7/1/01: Results of the previous day were reported and evaluated. Patient was scheduled for cardiac catheterization.

ECG Report: Mild ST and T-wave abnormalities suggest active ischemia. Normal sinus rhythm.

Treatment Plan:

Laboratory Tests Ordered: Cardiac profile
Other Tests Ordered: Cardiac catheterization

7/2/01: Patient resting comfortably. Patient remained pain-free with current medications.

Cardiac Catheterization Report: Coronary angiography revealed coronary artery disease in two vessels. The left anterior descending had a 99 percent stenosis in the midsegment with thrombus present. The left circumflex coronary artery had mild luminal irregularities. The right coronary artery had a filling defect in the midsegment of approximately 70 percent severity and a 90 percent stenosis at the origin of the posterior descending artery branch.

Treatment Plan:

Laboratory Tests Ordered: Cardiac profile

7/3/01: Patient was returned to the cardiac catheterization laboratory, at which time a rotational atherectomy of the mid left anterior descending coronary artery and mid right coronary artery was performed. The rotational atherectomy was successful on both lesions, reducing the 99 percent stenosis in the mid left anterior descending coronary artery to a 10 percent residual stenosis and reducing the 90 percent stenosis in the mid right coronary artery to no residual stenosis.

Treatment Plan:

Laboratory Tests Ordered: ABG, cardiac profile, CMP

7/4/01: Patient had an uneventful course post-percutaneous transluminal coronary angioplasty. He experienced no chest pain or arrhythmia, and his blood pressure remained in good control. Patient was advised on proper diet and exercise.

7/5/01: Patient has achieved maximum hospital benefit and was discharged with diagnoses of AMI and hyperlipidemia.

LEARNING ACTIVITIES

PATIENT: **Paul L. Richmond**
INSTRUCTIONS: *Before you begin, read the instructions carefully and follow each step in the process.*

STUDY GUIDES

Goal A

The goal in this activity is for you to relate laboratory data with Mr. Richmond's symptoms on his admission to the hospital. This learning activity will allow you to collect and assess initial data pertaining to Mr. Richmond.

Learning Issues

ISSUE 1: From the clinician's notes, identify relevant signs and symptoms, social and previous medical history, and results of the physical examination.

ISSUE 2: Identify significant laboratory findings that are related to Mr. Richmond's clinical condition at the time of presentation. Correlate these findings with his clinical presentation.

Issue 3: Review the laboratory test results provided in the documentation and correlate these data with Mr. Richmond's diagnoses.

Study Questions A

1. Review the patient's medical records and determine which of the presenting symptoms and which elements of the background history the physician may consider significant in his illness.

CLINICAL SYMPTOMS:

_____

_____

_____

_____

BACKGROUND HISTORY:

_____

_____

_____

_____

2. In the space provided, list the laboratory tests that were requested at the time of Mr. Richmond's admission. Which of the tests requested specifically correlate with his presenting symptoms? Highlight these tests.

_____

_____

_____

3. Now access the laboratory test results from the Laboratory Information System (LIS) in the CD-ROM. Obtain Mr. Richmond's results on admission and record them on the patient laboratory tests results forms provided in this workbook. Review Mr. Richmond's laboratory test results at the time he was admitted to the hospital.

   Note: If this is your first time accessing information in the CD-ROM, make sure that you start with "Before you begin."

4. a. Are any of the laboratory test results outside the usual acceptable range? List those results that are outside the usual acceptable range.

    b. Which laboratory test results indicate a cardiac problem?

    c. Are any of the results at critical levels?

    d. What do these results suggest?

5. Do these test results correlate with Mr. Richmond's presenting symptoms? How?

6. What are this patient's risk factors for cardiac disease?

7. What is the acid-base status of the patient on admission?

_____

_____

_____

_____

8. Is this state common for persons having an AMI? If so, why?

_____

_____

_____

_____

Goal B

In this portion of the learning activity, the goal is for you to evaluate follow-up measures taken during the course of Mr. Richmond's illness and how these measures relate to his prognosis and ultimate outcome. This learning activity will allow you to identify reasons for the requests for additional laboratory tests to be performed on this patient.

Learning Issues

ISSUE 1: Interpret the data collected on Mr. Richmond relating to treatment and prognosis.

ISSUE 2: Evaluate the use of the laboratory in this case.

Study Questions B

1. Describe the characteristic pattern of CK-MB elevations after a classic AMI.

_____

_____

_____

_____

2. Do Mr. Richmond's CK-MB results follow this pattern?

_____

_____

_____

_____

3. Describe the characteristic pattern of troponin I elevations after a classic AMI.

    _____

    _____

    _____

    _____

4. Do Mr. Richmond's troponin I results follow this pattern?

    _____

    _____

    _____

5. Why was the myoglobin concentration not followed as the CK-MB and troponin I elevations were followed?

    _____

    _____

    _____

6. Why was streptokinase or another clot-busting agent not administered to this patient on admission?

    _____

    _____

    _____

7. Why was a lipid profile ordered on admission?

    _____

    _____

    _____

8. Why is Mr. Richmond's white blood cell count elevated?

9. Discuss Mr. Richmond's decreased hemoglobin and hematocrit.

10. Are there any laboratory tests that have not been ordered on Mr. Richmond that would be helpful in arriving at a more specific diagnosis? If so, what tests do you think were omitted? *(This will be an individual response.)*

11. Discuss the appropriateness of the laboratory tests ordered on Mr. Richmond. Is the laboratory being overutilized or underutilized? Defend your answer. *(This will be an individual response.)*

UNIVERSITY MEDICAL CENTER

Name: _____   Date: _____

Record #: _____   Time: _____

ANTIBODY IDENTIFICATION PANEL

Vial	Special Type	Donor	Rh-Hr								Kell						Duffy		Kidd		Lewis		P	MN				Lutheran		Xg	Test Methods			
			D	C	c	E	e	f	V	Cw	K	k	Kp$_a$	Kp$_b$	Js$_a$	Js$_b$	Fy$_a$	Fy$_b$	Jk$_a$	Jk$_b$	Le$_a$	Le$_b$	P1	M	N	S	s	LU$_a$	LU$_b$	Xg$_a$	37	AGH	CC	
1	Bg(a+)	R1R1 B1080	+	+	0	0	+	0	0	0	0	+	0	+	0	+	+	0	0	+	0	+	+	+	+	+	+	0	+	+				1
2		R1WR1 B1102	+	+	0	0	+	0	0	+	0	+	0	+	0	+	0	+	+	+	0	+	+	0	0	0	+	0	+	0				2
3	Bg(a+)	R2R2 C1243	+	0	+	+	0	0	0	0	0	+	0	+	0	+	+	+	0	+	0	+	+	+	0	+	+	0	+	+				3
4		ROR D575	+	0	+	0	+	+	0	0	0	+	0	+	0	+	0	0	+	0	0	0	+	0	+	0	+	0	+	+				4
5		r'r E370	0	+	+	0	+	+	0	0	0	+	0	+	0	+	+	+	0	+	0	+	+	+	+	+	+	0	+	0				5
6		r"r F416	0	0	+	+	+	+	0	0	0	+	0	+	0	+	0	+	+	+	+	0	0	+	+	0	+	+	+	+				6
7		rrK G488	0	0	+	0	+	+	0	0	+	+	0	+	0	+	+	0	+	0	+	0	+	+	0	0	+	0	+	0				7
8	Yt(b+)	rrFya H347	0	0	+	0	+	+	0	0	0	+	0	+	0	+	+	+	0	+	0	+	+	+	+	+	+	0	+	0				8
9		rr N1434	0	0	+	0	+	+	0	0	0	+	0	+	0	+	+	+	+	+	+	0	+	+	0	+	0	0	+	+				9
10	Co(b+)	R2R2 C199	+	0	+	+	0	0	0	0	0	+	0	+	0	+	+	+	0	+	0	+	0	+	0	0	+	0	+	+				10
TC	He+	R1R2 A1086	+	+	+	+	+	0	0	0	0	+	0	+	0	+	+	0	+	+	0	+	+	+	+	+	+	+	+	0				TC
		Patient's Cells																																	

UNIVERSITY MEDICAL CENTER

Name: _____

Date: _____

Record #: _____

Time: _____

Cell Tests

Anti-A _____

Anti-B _____

Anti-D IS _____

Anti-D 37 _____

Anti-D AHG _____

Anti-A_1 Lectin _____

Serum Tests

	RT	37	AHG	CC
A_1 Cells	_____			
A_2 Cells	_____			
B Cells	_____			
Screen Cells I	_____	_____	_____	_____
Screen Cells II	_____	_____	_____	_____
Screen Cells III	_____	_____	_____	_____

UNIVERSITY MEDICAL CENTER
CONFIDENTIAL PATIENT INFORMATION
CUMULATIVE SUMMARY REPORT

PATIENT INFORMATION   ID number: _____   Ward: _____

Name: _____   Physician: _____

Address: _____   Date Admitted: _____

_____   Phone: _____

City: _____   State: _____   Zip: _____

Date of Birth: _____   Sex: _____   Race: _____

CHEMISTRY

Tests	Reference Ranges	Date: Time:	Date: Time:	Date: Time:	Date: Time:	Date: Time:
Acid Phos	2.5–11.7 U/L					
ACTH	9–52 pg/mL					
ALT	0–45 IU/L					
Albumin	3.5–5.0 g/dL					
A/G Ratio	0.7–2.1					
Aldosterone	??					
Alkaline Phos	41–137 IU/L					
Ammonia	11–35 µmol/L					
Amylase	95–290 U/L					
Anion Gap	10–18 mmol/L					
AST	0–41 IU/L					
Bilirubin	0.2–1.0 mg/dL					
Bilirubin (direct)	0.2–1.0 mg/dL					
BUN	10–20 mg/dL					
Calcium (total)	4.3–5.3 mEq/L					
Calcuim (ionized)	1.16–1.32 mmol/L					
Chloride	95–100 mmol/L					
Carbon Dioxide	23–32 mmol/L					

CHEMISTRY (page 2)

Tests	Reference Ranges	Date: Time:	Date: Time:	Date: Time:	Date: Time:	Date: Time:
Cholesterol	<200 mg/dL					
CK	15–160 U/L					
CK-MB	15–160 U/L					
Creatinine	0.7–1.5 mg/dL					
Creatintine Clearance	80–120 mL/min					
GGT	6–45 U/L					
Globulin	2.3–3.2 g/dL					
Glucose	65–105 mg/dL					
LD	100–225 U/L					
LDL Cholesterol	75–140 U/L					
LDL/HDL	2.9–2.2					
Lipase	0–1.0 U/mL					
Magnesium	1.3–2.1 mEq/L					
Osmolality	275–295 mOsM/kg					
Phosphorus	2.7–4.5 mg/dL					
Potassium	3.5–5.0 mmol/L					
Protein	5.8–8.2 g/dL					
Sodium	135–145 mmol/L					
Triglycerides	10–190 mg/dL					
Uric Acid	3.5–7.2 mg/dL					
HCO_3	100–225 U/L					

PATIENT INFORMATION   ID number: _____   Ward: _____

Name: _____   Physician: _____

Address: _____   Date Admitted: _____

_____   Phone: _____

City: _____   State: _____   Zip: _____

Date of Birth: _____   Sex: _____   Race: _____

HEMATOLOGY

Test	Reference Ranges	Date: Time:	Date: Time:	Date: Time:	Date: Time:	Date: Time:
Hemoglobin (g/dL) Male Female	14.0–18.0 12.0–15.0					
Hematocrit (%) Male Female	40–54 35–49					
RBC ($\times 10^{12}$/L) Male Female	4.6–6.6 4.0–5.4					
WBC ($\times 10^{9}$/L)	4.5–11.5					
MCV (fL)	80–94					
MCHC (g/dL or %)	32–36					
MCH (pg)	26–32					
Platelet Count ($\times 10^{9}$/L)	150–450					
RDW (%)	11.5–14.5					
Reticulocyte Count						
Segmented Neutrophils (%)	50–70					
Lymphocytes (%)	18–42					
Monocytes (%)	2–11					
Basophils (%)	0–2					
Eosinophils (%)	1–3					
Erythrocyte Sed Rate (ESR) Male Female	0–9 mm/hr 0–15 mm/hr					
Prothrombin Time (PT)	<2-sec deviation from control; 12–14 sec					
Activated Partial Thromboplastin Time (APTT)	<35 sec					
Fibrin Degradation Products (FDP)	4.9 ± 2.8 µg FDP/mL					
Thrombin Time	15 sec					
D-Dimer	<0.5 µg/mL					

UNIVERSITY MEDICAL CENTER

CONFIDENTIAL PATIENT INFORMATION
CUMULATIVE SUMMARY REPORT

PATIENT INFORMATION   ID number: _____   Ward: _____

Name: _____   Physician: _____

Address: _____   Date Admitted: _____

_____   Phone: _____

City: _____   State: _____   Zip: _____

Date of Birth: _____   Sex: _____   Race: _____

MICROBIOLOGY

Date and Time	Procedure / Specimen	Direct Smear	Preliminary Report	Final Report

CASE SUMMARY

A. Provide a brief summary of possible patient outcomes based on the laboratory test results and the patient's diagnoses.

_____
_____
_____
_____
_____
_____
_____
_____

B. Identify the learning points that you consider helpful in working up this patient's case. *(This will be an individual response.)*

_____
_____
_____
_____
_____
_____
_____
_____
_____

NOTES

_____
_____
_____
_____
_____
_____
_____
_____

► PATIENT'S RECORDS

PATIENT NAME: **Walter Roberts**

PATIENT IDENTIFICATION NUMBER: **246810**

PHYSICIAN: **James**

PATIENT INFORMATION

NAME: Walter Roberts   ID NUMBER: 246810

PHYSICIAN: James

DATE ADMITTED: 7/20/99   TIME: 1435

ADDRESS: 5248 Lexington Circle, Hillsdale, TN 38127

PHONE: 901-555-5316

DATE OF BIRTH: 3/30/60   SEX: M   RACE: W

ADMISSION INFORMATION

WT.: 210   HT.: 6'0"   B/P: 140/98

R: 30 unlabored   PULSE: 80   TEMP.: 99

MEDICATION: No prescribed meds; self-administered extra-strength Tylenol

ADMISSION DIAGNOSIS
Nausea, vomiting of unknown origin

PRIMARY COMPLAINT
Two-day history of severe nausea, vomiting, and weakness

PATIENT HISTORY

The patient is a 39-year-old white male with no significant past medical history except severe nausea and vomiting for the past 2 days. Physical examination is unremarkable except for moderate scleral icterus. The patient has a history of chronic headaches and self-medicates with Tylenol, taking 4 to 10 extra-strength Tylenol every day throughout the past year. Alcohol consumption consists of three or four rum-and-Cokes routinely on weekday evenings, with a higher intake on weekends. Within the past 2 weeks patient has participated in a half-court basketball game without undue fatigue. Patient denies any recent myalgias or arthralgias and states that he was completely well until 48 h prior to admission. Patient denies any known exposure to persons with hepatitis.

TREATMENT PLAN

Laboratory Tests Ordered: CBC, UA, CMP, PT, APTT, liver/spleen scan

PROGRESS REPORTS

7/20/99: Patient remained in ED awaiting laboratory results. The patient was admitted to the ICU with IV fluids and Phenergan to control nausea and vomiting. He received 2 units of FFP and 20 mg vitamin K in IV fluids. Urine output was quite small (140 mL).

Treatment Plan: Monitor patient's physical and mental status closely. Nephrology and hepatology consults ordered.

7/21/99: 20 mg vitamin K administered IV. Liver/renal function laboratory results monitored. Patient's mental status was altered and monitored closely.

Treatment Plan:

Laboratory Tests Ordered: UA, CMP, hepatitis profile, PT, PTT
Other Tests Ordered: Head MRI

7/21/99: Hepatology Consult Report:

Markedly abnormal liver parameters consistent with acute hepatocellular necrosis/fulminant liver failure. Initial liver/spleen scan showed fairly good liver function with good visualization of liver and some increased uptake in the spleen.

Treatment Plan: Monitor liver functions and coagulation parameters closely.

7/21/99: Nephrology Consult Report:

Rule out analgesic nephropathy with acute insult related to volume concentration. Papillary necrosis possible. Hydration OK.

Treatment Plan: Offer dialysis if necessary.

7/22/99: Renal dialysis was initiated in response to increasing BUN and creatinine. Neurologic consult was obtained with reference to patient's initial complaint of chronic headache. An MRI of the head was obtained, which was normal with the exception of several small areas of increased signal in the deep quiet matter that were difficult to interpret in light of the renal/liver failure and associated problems. The liver transplant team was consulted because of the severe nature of the liver insult and superior hepatocellular necrosis.

Treatment Plan:

Laboratory Tests Ordered: BUN, Cr, AST, ALT, total bilirubin, Cr clearance, PT, PTT

7/23/99: Urine output increased after dialysis, with improvements in BUN and creatinine concentrations. Patient was transferred from the ICU to a regular floor.

Treatment Plan:

Laboratory Tests Ordered: BUN, Cr, AST, ALT, total bilirubin

7/24/99–7/30/99: Patient continued to slowly improve both liver and renal functions. Patient's mental status continued to be good.

Treatment Plan:

Laboratory Tests Ordered:
  7/24/99: BUN, Cr, AST, ALT, total bilirubin, Cr clearance
  7/25/99: BUN, Cr, AST, ALT, total bilirubin
  7/26/99: BUN, Cr, AST, ALT, total bilirubin
  7/28/99: ALT
  7/30/99: ALT

7/31/99–8/1/99: Creatinine clearance much improved; liver function studies returning to normal.

Treatment Plan:

Laboratory Tests Ordered:
  7/31/99: BUN, Cr, Cr clearance, ALT
  8/1/99: BUN, Cr, ALT

8/2/99: Patient discharged in much improved condition, to be followed as an outpatient by nephrology for follow-up of renal function, by hepatology for reevaluation of liver status, and by neurology with regard to recurrence of headaches.

Treatment Plan:

Laboratory Tests Ordered: CBC, CMP
Discharge Diagnosis:
  1. Fulminant hepatic failure secondary to #3
  2. Acute renal failure secondary to #3

3. Chronic Tylenol/alcohol abuse
4. Tension headaches

LEARNING ACTIVITIES

PATIENT: **Walter Roberts**

INSTRUCTIONS: *Before you begin, read the instructions carefully and follow each step in the process.*

STUDY GUIDES

Goal A

The goal in this activity is for you to relate laboratory data with Mr. Roberts' symptoms, history, diagnosis, and prognosis on his admission to the hospital. This learning activity will allow you to collect and assess initial data pertaining to Mr. Roberts.

Learning Issues

ISSUE 1: From the clinician's notes, identify relevant signs and symptoms, social and previous medical history, and results of the physical examination.

ISSUE 2: Identify significant laboratory findings that are related to Mr. Roberts's clinical condition at the time of this admission. Correlate these findings with his clinical presentation.

ISSUE 3: Review the laboratory test results provided in the documentation and correlate these data with Mr. Roberts's diagnoses.

Study Questions A

1. Review the patient's medical records and determine which of the presenting symptoms and which elements of the background history the physician may consider significant in his current illness.

CLINICAL SYMPTOMS:

_____

_____

_____

_____

BACKGROUND HISTORY:

2. In the space provided, list the laboratory tests that were requested at the time of Mr. Roberts's admission. Which of the tests requested provide valuable information in the evaluation of his presenting symptoms? Highlight these tests.

3. Now access the laboratory test results from the Laboratory Information System (LIS) in the CD-ROM. Obtain Mr. Roberts's results and record them on the patient laboratory tests results forms provided in this workbook. Review Mr. Roberts's laboratory test results on the day of his admission.

   Note: If this is your first time accessing information in the CD-ROM, make sure that you start with "Before you begin."

4. a. Which of the several laboratory test results that fall outside the acceptable range indicate a renal problem?

   b. Which laboratory test results indicate a hepatic problem? If so, which ones?

c. Are any of the laboratory test results at critical levels?

d. What do these results suggest?

5. Do these test result correlate with Mr. Roberts's presenting symptoms? If so, how?

6. The results on Mr. Roberts indicate a renal problem. Which of the admission laboratory test results is most indicative of his renal failure?

7. Define clearance and show the formula for calculating creatinine clearance.

8. What is the purpose of a creatinine clearance evaluation?

Goal B

In this portion of the learning activity, the goal is for you to evaluate follow-up measures taken during the course of Mr. Roberts's illness and how these measures relate to his prognosis and ultimate outcome. This learning activity will allow you to identify reasons for the requests for additional laboratory tests to be performed on this patient.

Learning Issues

ISSUE 1: Interpret the data collected on Mr. Roberts relating to treatment and prognosis.

ISSUE 2: Evaluate the use of the laboratory in this case.

Study Questions B

1. Mr. Roberts had three creatinine clearance tests performed while in the hospital. What do the creatinine clearance test results suggest for this patient?

2. At what concentration does the serum creatinine value become critical? When did Mr. Roberts's value reach this critical point?

3. What is the cause of this patient's renal failure?

4. Discuss the effects of Tylenol/alcohol abuse on the kidneys.

5. Mr. Roberts's results also indicate a hepatic problem.

   a. Which laboratory results are most indicative of the severity of Mr. Roberts's liver failure?

   b. What are the common causes of liver failure?

   c. Why was an acetaminophen level not done on this patient at admission?

6. Why was fresh frozen plasma and vitamin K treatment started immediately on Mr. Roberts's admission to the ICU?

7. Mr. Roberts's discharge diagnosis noted that the hepatic and renal failure were secondary to chronic Tylenol (acetaminophen)/alcohol abuse.

   a. What are the symptoms of acetaminophen poisoning?

   _____

   _____

   _____

   _____

   b. What is the preferred treatment for acute acetaminophen poisoning?

   _____

   _____

   _____

   _____

   c. Why was this treatment not used for this patient?

   _____

   _____

   _____

   _____

   d. What is the treatment for chronic acetaminophen poisoning?

   _____

   _____

   _____

   _____

   e. Discuss the effects of acetaminophen/alcohol overdose on the liver.

   _____

   _____

   _____

   _____

8. Are there any laboratory tests that have not been ordered on Mr. Roberts that would be helpful in arriving at a more specific diagnosis? If so, what tests do you think were omitted?

9. Discuss the appropriateness of the laboratory tests ordered on Mr. Roberts. Is the laboratory being overutilized or underutilized? Defend your answer.

UNIVERSITY MEDICAL CENTER

Name: _____   Date: _____

Record #: _____   Time: _____

ANTIBODY IDENTIFICATION PANEL

Vial	Special Type	Donor	D	C	c	E	e	f	V	Cw	K	k	Kpa	Kpb	Jsa	Jsb	Fya	Fyb	Jka	Jkb	Lea	Leb	P1	M	N	S	s	LUa	LUb	Xga		37	AGH	CC
								Rh-Hr						Kell				Duffy		Kidd		Lewis		P		MN			Lutheran		Xg		Test Methods		
1	Bg(a+)	R1R1 B1080	+	+	0	0	+	0	0	0	0	+	0	+	0	+	+	0	0	+	0	+	+	+	+	+	+	0	+	+	1			
2		R1WR1 B1102	+	+	0	0	+	0	0	+	+	+	0	+	0	+	0	+	0	+	0	+	+	0	+	0	+	0	+	0	2			
3	Bg(a+)	R2R2 C1243	+	0	+	+	0	0	0	0	0	+	0	+	0	+	+	+	+	0	0	+	+	+	0	+	+	0	+	+	3			
4		ROR D575	+	0	+	0	+	+	0	0	0	+	0	+	0	+	0	0	0	+	0	0	+	+	+	0	+	0	+	+	4			
5		r'r E370	0	+	+	0	+	+	0	0	0	+	0	+	0	+	+	+	0	+	0	+	+	+	+	+	+	0	+	0	5			
6		r"r F416	0	0	+	+	+	+	0	0	0	+	0	+	0	+	+	+	+	+	+	0	0	+	+	0	+	+	+	+	6			
7		rrK G488	0	0	+	0	+	+	0	0	+	+	0	+	0	+	0	+	+	0	+	0	0	+	0	0	+	0	+	0	7			
8	Yt(b+)	rrFya H347	0	0	+	0	+	+	0	0	0	+	0	+	0	+	+	0	+	0	0	+	+	+	+	+	+	0	+	0	8			
9		rr N1434	0	0	+	0	+	+	0	0	0	+	0	+	0	+	+	+	+	0	0	0	+	0	+	0	0	0	+	+	9			
10	Co(b+)	R2R2 C199	+	0	+	+	0	0	0	0	0	+	0	+	0	+	+	+	+	0	+	0	0	+	+	0	+	0	+	+	10			
TC	He+	R1R2 A1086	+	+	+	+	+	+	0	0	0	+	0	+	0	+	0	+	0	0	0	+	+	+	+	+	+	+	+	0	TC			
		Patient's Cells																																

UNIVERSITY MEDICAL CENTER

Name: _____

Record #: _____

Date: _____

Time: _____

Cell Tests

Anti-A _____

Anti-B _____

Anti-D IS _____

Anti-D 37 _____

Anti-D AHG _____

Anti-A_1 Lectin _____

Serum Tests

	RT	37	AHG	CC
A_1 Cells	___			
A_2 Cells	___			
B Cells	___			
Screen Cells I	___	___	___	___
Screen Cells II	___	___	___	___
Screen Cells III	___	___	___	___

UNIVERSITY MEDICAL CENTER
CONFIDENTIAL PATIENT INFORMATION
CUMULATIVE SUMMARY REPORT

PATIENT INFORMATION   ID number: _____   Ward: _____

Name: _____   Physician: _____

Address: _____   Date Admitted: _____

_____   Phone: _____

City: _____   State: _____   Zip: _____

Date of Birth: _____   Sex: _____   Race: _____

CHEMISTRY

Tests	Reference Ranges	Date: Time:	Date: Time:	Date: Time:	Date: Time:	Date: Time:
Acid Phos	2.5–11.7 U/L					
ACTH	9–52 pg/mL					
ALT	0–45 IU/L					
Albumin	3.5–5.0 g/dL					
A/G Ratio	0.7–2.1					
Aldosterone	??					
Alkaline Phos	41–137 IU/L					
Ammonia	11–35 μmol/L					
Amylase	95–290 U/L					
Anion Gap	10–18 mmol/L					
AST	0–41 IU/L					
Bilirubin	0.2–1.0 mg/dL					
Bilirubin (direct)	0.2–1.0 mg/dL					
BUN	10–20 mg/dL					
Calcium (total)	4.3–5.3 mEq/L					
Calcuim (ionized)	1.16–1.32 mmol/L					
Chloride	95–100 mmol/L					
Carbon Dioxide	23–32 mmol/L					

CHEMISTRY (page 2)

Tests	Reference Ranges	Date: Time:	Date: Time:	Date: Time:	Date: Time:	Date: Time:
Cholesterol	<200 mg/dL					
CK	15–160 U/L					
CK-MB	15–160 U/L					
Creatinine	0.7–1.5 mg/dL					
Creatintine Clearance	80–120 mL/min					
GGT	6–45 U/L					
Globulin	2.3–3.2 g/dL					
Glucose	65–105 mg/dL					
LD	100–225 U/L					
LDL Cholesterol	75–140 U/L					
LDL/HDL	2.9–2.2					
Lipase	0–1.0 U/mL					
Magnesium	1.3–2.1 mEq/L					
Osmolality	275–295 mOsM/kg					
Phosphorus	2.7–4.5 mg/dL					
Potassium	3.5–5.0 mmol/L					
Protein	5.8–8.2 g/dL					
Sodium	135–145 mmol/L					
Triglycerides	10–190 mg/dL					
Uric Acid	3.5–7.2 mg/dL					
HCO_3	100–225 U/L					

PATIENT INFORMATION   ID number: _____   Ward: _____

Name: _____   Physician: _____

Address: _____   Date Admitted: _____

_____   Phone: _____

City: _____   State: _____   Zip: _____

Date of Birth: _____   Sex: _____   Race: _____

HEMATOLOGY

Test	Reference Ranges	Date: Time:	Date: Time:	Date: Time:	Date: Time:	Date: Time:

Hemoglobin (g/dL)
  Male
  Female
	14.0–18.0
	12.0–15.0					

Hematocrit (%)
  Male
  Female
	40–54
	35–49					

RBC ($\times 10^{12}$/L)
  Male
  Female
	4.6–6.6
	4.0–5.4					

WBC ($\times 10^{9}$/L)	4.5–11.5					
MCV (fL)	80–94					
MCHC (g/dL or %)	32–36					
MCH (pg)	26–32					
Platelet Count ($\times 10^{9}$/L)	150–450					
RDW (%)	11.5–14.5					
Reticulocyte Count						
Segmented Neutrophils (%)	50–70					
Lymphocytes (%)	18–42					
Monocytes (%)	2–11					
Basophils (%)	0–2					
Eosinophils (%)	1–3					

Erythrocyte Sed Rate (ESR)
  Male
  Female
	0–9 mm/hr
	0–15 mm/hr					

Prothrombin Time (PT)	<2-sec deviation from control; 12–14 sec					
Activated Partial Thromboplastin Time (APTT)	<35 sec					
Fibrin Degradation Products (FDP)	4.9 ± 2.8 µg FDP/mL					
Thrombin Time	15 sec					
D-Dimer	<0.5 µg/mL					

UNIVERSITY MEDICAL CENTER
CONFIDENTIAL PATIENT INFORMATION
CUMULATIVE SUMMARY REPORT

PATIENT INFORMATION   ID number: _____   Ward: _____

Name: _____   Physician: _____

Address: _____   Date Admitted: _____

_____   Phone: _____

City: _____   State: _____   Zip: _____

Date of Birth: _____   Sex: _____   Race: _____

MICROBIOLOGY

Date and Time	Procedure / Specimen	Direct Smear	Preliminary Report	Final Report

CASE SUMMARY

A. Provide a brief summary of possible patient outcomes based on the laboratory test results and the patient's progress.

_____
_____
_____
_____
_____
_____
_____

B. Identify the learning points that you consider helpful in working up this patient's case. *(This will be an individual response.)*

_____
_____
_____
_____
_____
_____
_____

NOTES

_____
_____
_____
_____
_____
_____
_____
_____

► PATIENT'S RECORDS

PATIENT NAME: **Aaron Shapely**

PATIENT IDENTIFICATION NUMBER: **789100**

PHYSICIAN: **Herrepin**

PATIENT INFORMATION

NAME: Aaron Shapely   ID NUMBER: 789100

PHYSICIAN: Herrepin

DATE ADMITTED: 2/3/00   TIME: 1300

ADDRESS: 1103 Cherry Dr., Manassas, VA 12389

PHONE: 703-555-1234

DATE OF BIRTH: 3/15/46   SEX: M   RACE: W

ADMISSION INFORMATION

WT.: 110 lb   HT.: 6'1"   B/P: 120/70

R: 24   PULSE: 84   TEMP: 101.2

ADMISSION DIAGNOSIS

Pneumonia

PRIMARY COMPLAINT

Cough, fever

PATIENT HISTORY

This patient is a 53-year-old white male patient who was seen at the clinic for an annual physical. The patient had complaints of a productive cough, fever, night sweats, and unexplained weight loss. The patient had been diagnosed as HIV positive 4 months previously, although he had not presented with any manifestations. He also had a history of chronic hepatitis B and intermittent oral herpes. He lived on a ranch, where he took care of farm animals. Two months prior to this admission, the patient had seen his personal physician, was diagnosed with bronchitis, and was unsuccessfully treated with Augmentin. Physical examination showed skin discolorations. A skin biopsy was taken, and a chest x-ray was requested. Lung tissue biopsies, skin biopsies, and blood and sputum cultures were also requested.

The patient was admitted for observation.

TREATMENT PLAN

Radiology: Chest x-ray revealed a large upper lobe infiltrate with cavitation formation.

Laboratory Tests Requested: Blood culture × 3; sputum bacterial, acid-fast bacilli (AFB), fungal cultures; lung tissue culture for bacteria, AFB, fungi; smear for *Pneumocystis carinii*

PROGRESS REPORTS

2/5/00, 1800: Patient remained stable. Cough and fever persisted. Loss of appetite.

Treatment Plan: Evaluate lab results. Request lymphocyte analysis (CD4/CD8 ratio). IV vancomycin started.

2/6/00, 1000: Skin biopsy pathology report confirmed positive for Kaposi sarcoma.

Lung biopsy smears reported negative for bacterial pathogens, parasites, or fungal agents. Culture results pending.

Treatment Plan: Repeat blood cultures.

2/7/00, 0600: The patient has remained stable. Diminished temperature.

First set of blood culture results showed positive; sputum culture positive.

Treatment Plan: Continue vancomycin; add erythromycin, ofloxacin, rifampin.

2/10/00, 0900: Second set of blood cultures positive.

Treatment Plan: Repeat blood cultures.

2/12/00, 0700: Fever has subsided. Additional blood cultures (third set) produced no growth. Patient is to be discharged from the hospital with a long-term antimicrobial therapy.

LEARNING ACTIVITIES

PATIENT: Aaron Shapely

INSTRUCTIONS: *Before you begin, read the instructions carefully and follow each step in the process.*

STUDY GUIDES

Goal A

The goal in this activity is for you to relate laboratory data with Mr. Shapely's symptoms on his admission to the hospital. This learning activity will allow you to collect and assess initial data pertaining to Mr. Shapely.

Learning Issues

ISSUE 1: Identify factors in his history that predispose Mr. Shapely to his condition.

ISSUE 2: Identify the significance of this information for your attempt to determine the etiology of his condition.

Study Questions A

1. Review the patient's medical records and determine which of the presenting symptoms and which elements of the background history the physician may consider significant in his illness.

CLINICAL SYMPTOMS:

_____

_____

_____

_____

BACKGROUND HISTORY:

_____

_____

_____

_____

2. In the space provided, list the laboratory tests that were requested at the time of Mr. Shapely's admission to the facility. Which of the tests requested specifically correlate with his presenting symptoms? Highlight these tests.

3. Now access the laboratory test results from the Laboratory Information System (LIS) in the CD-ROM. Obtain Mr. Shapely's results and record them on the patient laboratory test results forms provided in this workbook. Review Mr. Shapely's laboratory test results at the time he was admitted to the hospital.

    Note: If this is your first time accessing information in the CD-ROM, make sure that you start with "Before you begin."

4. a. Are any of the laboratory test results outside the usual acceptable range? If so, what do these results suggest?

    b. How do these test results correlate with Mr. Shapely's presenting symptoms?

5. Are there other laboratory findings that you consider significant in this case, given the background history of the patient?

Goal B

In this portion of the learning activity, the goal is for you to evaluate the patient's laboratory test results and determine how these results relate to his prognosis and ultimate outcome.

Learning Issues

ISSUE 1: Determine why the lymphocyte profile results are significant parameters in monitoring this disease process.

ISSUE 2: Consider the significance of the request to examine tissue samples for *Pneumocystis carinii.*

Study Questions B

1. Access the LIS on the CD-ROM for the identification of the organisms isolated from the sputum and blood cultures. Use the microbiology laboratory worksheets provided in this workbook to record the microscopic findings, biochemical tests performed, appropriate results, and identification of the organism(s). Evaluate the results. What organism(s) was (were) isolated from the blood and sputum cultures?

   _____

   _____

   _____

   _____

2. a. What errors may be made in identifying this particular isolate?

   _____

   _____

   _____

   _____

   b. How can this be prevented?

   _____

   _____

   _____

   _____

3. Why is this patient particularly susceptible to this type of pulmonary disease?

4. Why is finding *Pneumocystis carinii* in tissue samples significant?

UNIVERSITY MEDICAL CENTER

Name: _____ Date: _____

Record #: _____ Time: _____

ANTIBODY IDENTIFICATION PANEL

Vial	Special Type	Donor	D	C	c	E	e	f	V	Cw	K	k	Kpa	Kpb	Jsa	Jsb	Fya	Fyb	Jka	Jkb	Lea	Leb	P1	M	N	S	s	LUa	LUb	Xga	37	AGH	CC
							Rh-Hr							Kell			Duffy		Kidd		Lewis		P	MN				Lutheran		Xg	Test Methods		
1	Bg(a+)	R1R1 B1080	+	+	0	0	+	0	0	0	0	+	0	+	0	+	+	0	0	+	0	+	+	+	+	+	+	0	+	+			
2		R1WR1 B1102	+	+	0	0	+	0	0	+	+	+	0	+	0	+	0	+	+	+	0	+	+	0	+	0	+	0	+	0			
3	Bg(a+)	R2R2 C1243	+	0	+	+	0	0	0	0	0	+	0	+	0	+	+	+	+	0	0	0	+	+	0	+	+	0	+	+			
4		ROR D575	+	0	+	0	+	+	0	0	0	+	0	+	0	+	0	0	+	0	0	0	+	0	+	0	+	0	+	+			
5		r'r E370	0	+	+	0	+	+	0	0	0	+	0	+	0	+	+	0	0	+	0	0	+	+	+	+	+	0	+	0			
6		r"r F416	0	0	+	+	+	+	0	0	0	+	0	+	0	+	0	+	0	+	+	0	0	+	0	0	+	+	+	+			
7		rrK G488	0	0	+	0	+	+	0	0	+	0	0	+	0	+	0	0	0	+	+	0	0	+	0	0	+	0	+	0			
8	Yt(b+)	rrFya H347	0	0	+	0	+	+	0	0	0	+	0	+	0	+	+	0	+	+	+	0	+	+	+	+	+	0	+	0			
9		rr N1434	0	0	+	0	+	+	0	0	0	+	0	+	0	+	+	+	+	+	0	+	+	+	+	0	0	0	+	+			
10	Co(b+)	R2R2 C199	+	0	+	+	0	0	0	0	0	+	0	+	0	+	+	+	+	+	+	0	0	+	+	0	+	0	+	+			
TC	He+	R1R2 A1086	+	+	+	+	+	0	0	0	0	+	0	+	0	+	0	0	0	+	0	+	+	+	+	+	+	+	+	0			TC
		Patient's Cells																															

UNIVERSITY MEDICAL CENTER

Name: _____

Record #: _____

Date: _____

Time: _____

Cell Tests

Anti-A	_____
Anti-B	_____
Anti-D IS	_____
Anti-D 37	_____
Anti-D AHG	_____
Anti-A₁ Lectin	_____

Serum Tests

A₁ Cells	_____
A₂ Cells	_____
B Cells	_____

	RT	37	AHG	CC
Screen Cells I	___	___	___	___
Screen Cells II	___	___	___	___
Screen Cells III	___	___	___	___

UNIVERSITY MEDICAL CENTER

CONFIDENTIAL PATIENT INFORMATION
CUMULATIVE SUMMARY REPORT

PATIENT INFORMATION

ID number: _____ Ward: _____

Name: _____ Physician: _____

Address: _____ Date Admitted: _____

_____ Phone: _____

City: _____ State: _____ Zip: _____

Date of Birth: _____ Sex: _____ Race: _____

CHEMISTRY

Tests	Reference Ranges	Date: Time:	Date: Time:	Date: Time:	Date: Time:	Date: Time:
Acid Phos	2.5–11.7 U/L					
ACTH	9–52 pg/mL					
ALT	0–45 IU/L					
Albumin	3.5–5.0 g/dL					
A/G Ratio	0.7–2.1					
Aldosterone	??					
Alkaline Phos	41–137 IU/L					
Ammonia	11–35 μmol/L					
Amylase	95–290 U/L					
Anion Gap	10–18 mmol/L					
AST	0–41 IU/L					
Bilirubin	0.2–1.0 mg/dL					
Bilirubin (direct)	0.2–1.0 mg/dL					
BUN	10–20 mg/dL					
Calcium (total)	4.3–5.3 mEq/L					
Calcuim (ionized)	1.16–1.32 mmol/L					
Chloride	95–100 mmol/L					
Carbon Dioxide	23–32 mmol/L					

CHEMISTRY (page 2)

Tests	Reference Ranges	Date: Time:	Date: Time:	Date: Time:	Date: Time:	Date: Time:
Cholesterol	<200 mg/dL					
CK	15–160 U/L					
CK-MB	15–160 U/L					
Creatinine	0.7–1.5 mg/dL					
Creatintine Clearance	80–120 mL/min					
GGT	6–45 U/L					
Globulin	2.3–3.2 g/dL					
Glucose	65–105 mg/dL					
LD	100–225 U/L					
LDL Cholesterol	75–140 U/L					
LDL/HDL	2.9–2.2					
Lipase	0–1.0 U/mL					
Magnesium	1.3–2.1 mEq/L					
Osmolality	275–295 mOsM/kg					
Phosphorus	2.7–4.5 mg/dL					
Potassium	3.5–5.0 mmol/L					
Protein	5.8–8.2 g/dL					
Sodium	135–145 mmol/L					
Triglycerides	10–190 mg/dL					
Uric Acid	3.5–7.2 mg/dL					
HCO_3	100–225 U/L					

UNIVERSITY MEDICAL CENTER
CONFIDENTIAL PATIENT INFORMATION
CUMULATIVE SUMMARY REPORT

PATIENT INFORMATION   ID number: _____   Ward: _____

Name: _____   Physician: _____

Address: _____   Date Admitted: _____

_____   Phone: _____

City: _____   State: _____   Zip: _____

Date of Birth: _____   Sex: _____   Race: _____

HEMATOLOGY

Test	Reference Ranges	Date: Time:	Date: Time:	Date: Time:	Date: Time:	Date: Time:
Hemoglobin (g/dL)						
Male	14.0–18.0					
Female	12.0–15.0					
Hematocrit (%)						
Male	40–54					
Female	35–49					
RBC ($\times 10^{12}$/L)						
Male	4.6–6.6					
Female	4.0–5.4					
WBC ($\times 10^9$/L)	4.5–11.5					
MCV (fL)	80–94					
MCHC (g/dL or %)	32–36					
MCH (pg)	26–32					
Platelet Count ($\times 10^9$/L)	150–450					
RDW (%)	11.5–14.5					
Reticulocyte Count						
Segmented Neutrophils (%)	50–70					
Lymphocytes (%)	18–42					
Monocytes (%)	2–11					
Basophils (%)	0–2					
Eosinophils (%)	1–3					
Erythrocyte Sed Rate (ESR)						
Male	0–9 mm/hr					
Female	0–15 mm/hr					
Prothrombin Time (PT)	<2-sec deviation from control; 12–14 sec					
Activated Partial Thromboplastin Time (APTT)	<35 sec					
Fibrin Degradation Products (FDP)	4.9 ± 2.8 µg FDP/mL					
Thrombin Time	15 sec					
D-Dimer	<0.5 µg/mL					

UNIVERSITY MEDICAL CENTER
CONFIDENTIAL PATIENT INFORMATION
CUMULATIVE SUMMARY REPORT

PATIENT INFORMATION   ID number: _____   Ward: _____

Name: _____   Physician: _____

Address: _____   Date Admitted: _____

_____   Phone: _____

City: _____   State: _____   Zip: _____

Date of Birth: _____   Sex: _____   Race: _____

MICROBIOLOGY

Date and Time	Procedure / Specimen	Direct Smear	Preliminary Report	Final Report

CASE SUMMARY

A. Provide a brief summary of possible patient outcomes based on the laboratory test results and the patient's diagnoses.

_____

_____

_____

_____

_____

_____

_____

B. Identify the learning points that you consider helpful in working up this patient's case. *(This will be an individual response.)*

_____

_____

_____

_____

_____

_____

_____

_____

NOTES

_____

_____

_____

_____

_____

_____

_____

▶ PATIENT'S RECORDS

PATIENT NAME: **Jason Stewart**

PATIENT IDENTIFICATION NUMBER: **994294**

PHYSICIAN: **Monroe**

PATIENT INFORMATION

NAME: Jason Stewart   ID NUMBER: 994294

PHYSICIAN: Monroe

DATE ADMITTED: 2/25/02   TIME: 1200

ADDRESS: 5400 Georgia Ave., Cokeville, WV 13012

PHONE: 230-555-1212

DATE OF BIRTH: 03/15/30   SEX: M   RACE: W   WARD: 3S

ADMISSION INFORMATION

WT.: 130 lb   HT.: 6'1"   B/P: 102/70

R: 18   PULSE: 122   TEMP: 101.2

ADMISSION DIAGNOSIS

Anemia

PRIMARY COMPLAINT

Dysphasia

PATIENT HISTORY

The patient is a 72-year-old male who came to the health clinic complaining of dysphasia. No other medical or familial history was known at the time of patient presentation at the clinic. The patient was admitted for work-up and observation.

PHYSICAL EXAMINATION

His physical exam showed no signs of leukemia (fever, fatigue, weight loss) or any organ enlargement.

TREATMENT PLAN

Laboratory Test Ordered: CBC

PROGRESS REPORTS

Day 2, 1800: Patient was stable and seemed calm and oriented. Reviewed laboratory results. Initial diagnosis: Anemia, leukemia.

Treatment Plan: Request bone marrow biopsy. Request flow cytometry studies.

Day 4, 1000: Flow cytometry and bone marrow studies determined final diagnosis.

Treatment Plan: No chemotherapy or other treatment given at this time. Will discharge and follow up as an outpatient.

LEARNING ACTIVITIES

PATIENT: **Jason Stewart**
INSTRUCTIONS: *Before you begin, read the instructions carefully and follow each step in the process.*

STUDY GUIDES

Goal

The goal in this activity is for you to relate laboratory data with Mr. Stewart's symptoms on his admission to the hospital. This learning activity will allow you to collect and assess initial data pertaining to Mr. Stewart.

Learning Issues

Issue 1: Identify physical findings presented by Mr. Stewart that are considered typical for his diagnosed condition.

Issue 2: Determine the laboratory findings that are significant in the diagnosis of his condition.

Study Questions

1. Review the patient's medical records and determine which of the presenting symptoms and which elements of the background history the physician may consider significant in his illness.

CLINICAL SYMPTOMS:

_____

_____

_____

_____

BACKGROUND HISTORY:

_____

_____

_____

_____

2. In the space provided, list the laboratory tests that were requested at the time of Mr. Stewart's admission to the facility. Which of the tests requested specifically correlate with his presenting symptoms? Highlight these tests.

_____

_____

_____

_____

3. Now access the laboratory test results from the Laboratory Information System (LIS) in the CD-ROM. Obtain Mr. Stewart's results and record them on the patient laboratory tests results forms provided in this workbook. Review Mr. Stewart's laboratory test results at the time he was admitted to the hospital.

    Note: If this is your first time accessing information in the CD-ROM, make sure that you start with "Before you begin."

4. a. Are any of the laboratory test results outside the usual acceptable ranges? If so, what do these results suggest?

    b. What features observed on the peripheral blood and bone marrow smears are characteristic of Mr. Stewart's diagnosed condition?

5. Are there other laboratory findings that you consider significant in this case, given the background history of the patient (e.g., culture results)?

6. What diagnosis was made based on the clinical and laboratory findings?

7. a. How is the classification (staging) system of Mr. Stewart's condition defined? Based on his progress reports, what is the stage of Mr. Stewart's illness?

b. What is the prognosis of his condition?

_____

_____

_____

_____

UNIVERSITY MEDICAL CENTER

Name: _____ Date: _____

Record #: _____ Time: _____

ANTIBODY IDENTIFICATION PANEL

Vial	Special Type	Donor	D	C	c	E	e	f	V	Cw	K	k	Kpa	Kpb	Jsa	Jsb	Fya	Fyb	Jka	Jkb	Lea	Leb	P1	M	N	S	s	LUa	LUb	Xga	37	AGH	CC
							Rh-Hr						Kell				Duffy		Kidd		Lewis		P	MN				Lutheran		Xg	Test Methods		
1	Bg(a+)	R1R1 B1080	+	+	0	0	+	0	0	0	0	+	0	+	0	+	+	0	0	+	0	+	+	+	+	+	+	0	+	+	1		
2		R1WR1 B1102	+	+	0	0	+	0	0	+	+	+	0	+	0	+	0	+	+	+	0	+	+	0	+	0	+	0	+	0	2		
3	Bg(a+)	R2R2 C1243	+	0	+	+	0	0	0	0	0	+	0	+	0	+	+	+	0	+	0	0	+	+	0	+	+	0	+	+	3		
4		ROR D575	+	0	+	0	+	+	0	0	0	+	0	+	0	+	0	0	+	0	0	0	+	+	+	0	+	0	+	+	4		
5		r'r E370	0	+	+	0	+	+	0	0	0	+	0	+	0	+	+	+	0	0	0	+	+	+	+	+	+	0	+	0	5		
6		r"r F416	0	0	+	+	+	+	0	0	0	+	0	+	0	+	0	0	+	+	+	0	0	+	+	0	+	+	+	+	6		
7		rrK G488	0	0	+	0	+	+	0	0	+	+	0	+	0	+	0	0	0	0	+	0	0	+	0	0	+	0	+	0	7		
8	Yt(b+)	rrFya H347	0	0	+	0	+	+	0	0	0	+	0	+	0	+	+	0	+	0	+	0	+	+	+	+	0	0	+	0	8		
9		rr N1434	0	0	+	0	+	+	0	0	0	+	0	+	0	+	+	+	+	0	0	+	+	+	0	+	0	0	+	+	9		
10	Co(b+)	R2R2 C199	+	0	+	+	0	0	0	0	0	+	0	+	0	+	+	0	+	0	+	0	+	+	+	+	+	0	+	+	10		
TC	He+	R1R2 A1086	+	+	+	+	+	0	0	0	0	+	0	+	0	+	0	+	0	0	0	+	+	+	+	+	+	+	+	0	TC		
		Patient's Cells																															

UNIVERSITY MEDICAL CENTER

Name: _____

Record #: _____

Date: _____

Time: _____

Cell Tests

Anti-A _____

Anti-B _____

Anti-D IS _____

Anti-D 37 _____

Anti-D AHG _____

Anti-A$_1$ Lectin _____

Serum Tests

A$_1$ Cells _____

A$_2$ Cells _____

B Cells _____

	RT	37	AHG	CC
Screen Cells I	___	___	___	___
Screen Cells II	___	___	___	___
Screen Cells III	___	___	___	___

UNIVERSITY MEDICAL CENTER
CONFIDENTIAL PATIENT INFORMATION
CUMULATIVE SUMMARY REPORT

PATIENT INFORMATION   ID number: _____   Ward: _____

Name: _____   Physician: _____

Address: _____   Date Admitted: _____

_____   Phone: _____

City: _____   State: _____   Zip: _____

Date of Birth: _____   Sex: _____   Race: _____

CHEMISTRY

Tests	Reference Ranges	Date: Time:	Date: Time:	Date: Time:	Date: Time:	Date: Time:
Acid Phos	2.5–11.7 U/L					
ACTH	9–52 pg/mL					
ALT	0–45 IU/L					
Albumin	3.5–5.0 g/dL					
A/G Ratio	0.7–2.1					
Aldosterone	??					
Alkaline Phos	41–137 IU/L					
Ammonia	11–35 μmol/L					
Amylase	95–290 U/L					
Anion Gap	10–18 mmol/L					
AST	0–41 IU/L					
Bilirubin	0.2–1.0 mg/dL					
Bilirubin (direct)	0.2–1.0 mg/dL					
BUN	10–20 mg/dL					
Calcium (total)	4.3–5.3 mEq/L					
Calcuim (ionized)	1.16–1.32 mmol/L					
Chloride	95–100 mmol/L					
Carbon Dioxide	23–32 mmol/L					

CHEMISTRY (page 2)

Tests	Reference Ranges	Date: Time:	Date: Time:	Date: Time:	Date: Time:	Date: Time:
Cholesterol	<200 mg/dL					
CK	15–160 U/L					
CK-MB	15–160 U/L					
Creatinine	0.7–1.5 mg/dL					
Creatintine Clearance	80–120 mL/min					
GGT	6–45 U/L					
Globulin	2.3–3.2 g/dL					
Glucose	65–105 mg/dL					
LD	100–225 U/L					
LDL Cholesterol	75–140 U/L					
LDL/HDL	2.9–2.2					
Lipase	0–1.0 U/mL					
Magnesium	1.3–2.1 mEq/L					
Osmolality	275–295 mOsM/kg					
Phosphorus	2.7–4.5 mg/dL					
Potassium	3.5–5.0 mmol/L					
Protein	5.8–8.2 g/dL					
Sodium	135–145 mmol/L					
Triglycerides	10–190 mg/dL					
Uric Acid	3.5–7.2 mg/dL					
HCO_3	100–225 U/L					

UNIVERSITY MEDICAL CENTER
CONFIDENTIAL PATIENT INFORMATION
CUMULATIVE SUMMARY REPORT

PATIENT INFORMATION   ID number: _____   Ward: _____

Name: _____   Physician: _____

Address: _____   Date Admitted: _____

_____   Phone: _____

City: _____   State: _____   Zip: _____

Date of Birth: _____   Sex: _____   Race: _____

HEMATOLOGY

Test	Reference Ranges	Date: Time:	Date: Time:	Date: Time:	Date: Time:	Date: Time:
Hemoglobin (g/dL) Male Female	14.0–18.0 12.0–15.0					
Hematocrit (%) Male Female	40–54 35–49					
RBC (×10^{12}/L) Male Female	4.6–6.6 4.0–5.4					
WBC (×10^9/L)	4.5–11.5					
MCV (fL)	80–94					
MCHC (g/dL or %)	32–36					
MCH (pg)	26–32					
Platelet Count (×10^9/L)	150–450					
RDW (%)	11.5–14.5					
Reticulocyte Count						
Segmented Neutrophils (%)	50–70					
Lymphocytes (%)	18–42					
Monocytes (%)	2–11					
Basophils (%)	0–2					
Eosinophils (%)	1–3					
Erythrocyte Sed Rate (ESR) Male Female	0–9 mm/hr 0–15 mm/hr					
Prothrombin Time (PT)	<2-sec deviation from control; 12–14 sec					
Activated Partial Thromboplastin Time (APTT)	<35 sec					
Fibrin Degradation Products (FDP)	4.9 ± 2.8 µg FDP/mL					
Thrombin Time	15 sec					
D-Dimer	<0.5 µg/mL					

UNIVERSITY MEDICAL CENTER
CONFIDENTIAL PATIENT INFORMATION
CUMULATIVE SUMMARY REPORT

PATIENT INFORMATION   ID number: _____   Ward: _____

Name: _____   Physician: _____

Address: _____   Date Admitted: _____

_____   Phone: _____

City: _____   State: _____   Zip: _____

Date of Birth: _____   Sex: _____   Race: _____

MICROBIOLOGY

Date and Time	Procedure / Specimen	Direct Smear	Preliminary Report	Final Report

CASE SUMMARY

A. Provide a brief summary of possible patient outcomes based on the laboratory test results and the patient's diagnoses.

_____

_____

_____

_____

_____

_____

_____

_____

B. Identify the learning points that you consider helpful in working up this patient's case. *(This will be an individual response.)*

_____

_____

_____

_____

_____

_____

_____

_____

_____

NOTES

_____

_____

_____

_____

_____

_____

_____

_____

_____

► PATIENT'S RECORDS

PATIENT NAME: **Irma Van Heusen**

PATIENT IDENTIFICATION NUMBER: **132051**

PHYSICIAN: **Archey**

PATIENT INFORMATION

NAME: Irma Van Heusen   ID NUMBER: 132051

PHYSICIAN: Archey

DATE ADMITTED: 1/2/00   TIME: 0800

ADDRESS: 350 Deday St., Arlington, VA 20301

PHONE: 703-555-2221

DATE OF BIRTH: 3/31/35   SEX: F   RACE: W   WARD: 3E

ADMISSION INFORMATION

WT.: 145 lb   HT.: 5'3"   B/P: 100/60

R: 24   PULSE: 102   TEMP.: 102

ANTIBIOTICS TAKEN:

ADMISSION DIAGNOSIS
Bacteremia/sepsis

PRIMARY COMPLAINT
Fever, shortness of breath, nausea and vomiting, chills

PATIENT HISTORY

The patient is a 64-year-old white female who came to the hospital because of fever, shortness of breath, nausea, vomiting, rigor, and chills. The patient's clinical history included pacemaker insertion 10 days prior to this admission. Physical examination showed atrial fibrillation and mitral valve regurgitation. No other history is provided.0.

TREATMENT PLAN

Radiology Ordered: Chest x-ray
Laboratory Tests Ordered: Glucose, BUN, electrolytes, urinalysis, CBC, cardiac enzymes, blood cultures ×2

PROGRESS REPORTS

1/2/00, 2300: Blood culture reported viridans streptococci on the first set. Enterococci were isolated from set 2.

Treatment Plan: The patient was placed on gentamicin and penicillin.

1/4/00, 0800: Corrected report on blood culture set 1 was noted.

Treatment Plan: Repeat CBC and blood cultures.

1/6/00, 0800: Follow-up blood cultures were negative. Discharge patient with antibiotic prophylactic therapy.

LEARNING ACTIVITIES

PATIENT: Irma Van Heusen
INSTRUCTIONS: *Before you begin, read the instructions carefully and follow each step in the process.*

STUDY GUIDES

Goal A

The goal in this activity is for you to relate laboratory data with Ms. Van Heusen's symptoms on her admission to the hospital. This learning activity will allow you to collect and assess initial data pertaining to Ms. Van Heusen.

Learning Issues

ISSUE 1: Identify factors in her medical history that predispose Ms. Van Heusen to her condition.

ISSUE 2: Identify the significance of this information for your attempt to determine the etiology of her condition.

Study Questions A

1. Review the patient's medical records and determine which of the presenting symptoms and which elements of the background history the physician may consider significant in her illness.

CLINICAL SYMPTOMS:

_____

_____

_____

_____

BACKGROUND HISTORY:

_____

_____

_____

_____

2. In the space provided, list the laboratory tests that were requested at the time of Ms. Van Heusen's admission to the facility. Which of the tests requested specifically correlate with her presenting symptoms? Highlight these tests.

_____

_____

_____

_____

3. Now access the laboratory test results from the Laboratory Information System (LIS) in the CD-ROM. Obtain Ms. Van Heusen's results and record them on the patient laboratory tests results forms provided in this workbook. Review Ms. Van Heusen's laboratory test results at the time she was admitted to the hospital.

    Note: If this is your first time accessing information in the CD-ROM, make sure that you start with "Before you begin."

4. a. Are any of the laboratory test results outside the usual acceptable range? If so, what do these results suggest?

    _____

    _____

    _____

    _____

    b. How do these test results correlate with Ms. Van Heusen's presenting symptoms?

    _____

    _____

    _____

5. Are there other laboratory findings that you consider significant in this case, given the background history of the patient (e.g., culture results)?

    _____

    _____

    _____

    _____

Goal B

In this portion of the learning activity, the goal is for you to evaluate the patient's laboratory test results and determine how these results relate to her prognosis and ultimate outcome.

Learning Issues

ISSUE 1: Determine why the cardiac enzyme profile results are significant parameters in the diagnosis of this patient's disease process.

ISSUE 2: Consider the significance of the organisms isolated from the blood cultures.

Study Questions B

1. Access the LIS on the CD-ROM for the identification of the organisms isolated from the sputum and blood cultures. Use the microbiology laboratory worksheets provided in this workbook to record the microscopic findings, biochemical tests performed, appropriate results, and identification of the organism(s). What organism(s) was (were) isolated from the blood cultures?

2. How do these findings correlate with Ms. Van Heusen's background history?

3. What errors may be made in isolating and identifying this particular organism? What would be the consequences?

UNIVERSITY MEDICAL CENTER

Name: _____ Date: _____

Record #: _____ Time: _____

ANTIBODY IDENTIFICATION PANEL

Vial	Special Type	Donor	D	C	c	E	e	f	V	Cw	K	k	Kpa	Kpb	Jsa	Jsb	Fya	Fyb	Jka	Jkb	Lea	Leb	P1	M	N	S	s	LUa	LUb	Xga	37	AGH	CC	
1	Bg(a+)	R1R1 B1080	+	+	0	0	+	0	0	0	0	+	0	+	0	+	+	0	0	+	0	+	+	+	+	+	+	0	+	+				1
2		R1WR1 B1102	+	+	0	0	+	0	0	+	+	+	0	+	0	+	0	+	+	+	0	+	+	0	+	0	+	0	+	0				2
3	Bg(a+)	R2R2 C1243	+	0	+	+	0	0	0	0	0	+	0	+	0	+	+	+	+	0	0	+	+	+	0	+	+	0	+	+				3
4		ROR D575	+	0	+	0	+	+	0	0	0	+	0	+	0	+	0	0	+	0	0	0	+	+	+	0	+	0	+	+				4
5		r'r E370	0	+	+	0	+	+	0	0	0	+	0	+	0	+	0	+	0	+	0	+	+	+	+	+	+	0	+	0				5
6		r"r F416	0	0	+	+	+	+	0	0	0	+	0	+	0	+	0	+	+	+	0	+	+	+	+	0	+	+	+	+				6
7		rrK G488	0	0	+	0	+	+	0	0	+	+	0	+	0	+	0	+	0	+	+	0	0	+	0	0	+	0	+	0				7
8	Yt(b+)	rrFya H347	0	0	+	0	+	+	0	0	0	+	0	+	0	+	+	0	+	0	+	0	+	+	+	+	+	0	+	0				8
9		rr N1434	0	0	+	0	+	+	0	0	0	+	0	+	0	+	+	+	+	0	0	0	+	0	+	+	0	0	+	+				9
10	Co(b+)	R2R2 C199	+	0	+	+	0	0	0	0	0	+	0	+	0	+	+	+	0	0	+	0	0	+	+	+	+	0	+	+				10
TC	He+	R1R2 A1086	+	+	+	+	+	0	0	0	0	+	0	+	0	+	0	0	0	+	0	+	+	+	+	+	+	+	+	0				TC
		Patient's Cells																																

UNIVERSITY MEDICAL CENTER

Name: _____

Record #: _____

Date: _____

Time: _____

Cell Tests

Anti-A _____

Anti-B _____

Anti-D IS _____

Anti-D 37 _____

Anti-D AHG _____

Anti-A₁ Lectin _____

Serum Tests

	RT	37	AHG	CC
A₁ Cells	___			
A₂ Cells	___			
B Cells	___			
Screen Cells I	___	___	___	___
Screen Cells II	___	___	___	___
Screen Cells III	___	___	___	___

UNIVERSITY MEDICAL CENTER
CONFIDENTIAL PATIENT INFORMATION
CUMULATIVE SUMMARY REPORT

PATIENT INFORMATION   ID number: _____   Ward: _____

Name: _____   Physician: _____

Address: _____   Date Admitted: _____

_____   Phone: _____

City: _____   State: _____   Zip: _____

Date of Birth: _____   Sex: _____   Race: _____

CHEMISTRY

Tests	Reference Ranges	Date: Time:	Date: Time:	Date: Time:	Date: Time:	Date: Time:
Acid Phos	2.5–11.7 U/L					
ACTH	9–52 pg/mL					
ALT	0–45 IU/L					
Albumin	3.5–5.0 g/dL					
A/G Ratio	0.7–2.1					
Aldosterone	??					
Alkaline Phos	41–137 IU/L					
Ammonia	11–35 µmol/L					
Amylase	95–290 U/L					
Anion Gap	10–18 mmol/L					
AST	0–41 IU/L					
Bilirubin	0.2–1.0 mg/dL					
Bilirubin (direct)	0.2–1.0 mg/dL					
BUN	10–20 mg/dL					
Calcium (total)	4.3–5.3 mEq/L					
Calcuim (ionized)	1.16–1.32 mmol/L					
Chloride	95–100 mmol/L					
Carbon Dioxide	23–32 mmol/L					

CHEMISTRY (page 2)

Tests	Reference Ranges	Date: Time:	Date: Time:	Date: Time:	Date: Time:	Date: Time:
Cholesterol	<200 mg/dL					
CK	15–160 U/L					
CK-MB	15–160 U/L					
Creatinine	0.7–1.5 mg/dL					
Creatintine Clearance	80–120 mL/min					
GGT	6–45 U/L					
Globulin	2.3–3.2 g/dL					
Glucose	65–105 mg/dL					
LD	100–225 U/L					
LDL Cholesterol	75–140 U/L					
LDL/HDL	2.9–2.2					
Lipase	0–1.0 U/mL					
Magnesium	1.3–2.1 mEq/L					
Osmolality	275–295 mOsM/kg					
Phosphorus	2.7–4.5 mg/dL					
Potassium	3.5–5.0 mmol/L					
Protein	5.8–8.2 g/dL					
Sodium	135–145 mmol/L					
Triglycerides	10–190 mg/dL					
Uric Acid	3.5–7.2 mg/dL					
HCO_3	100–225 U/L					

PATIENT INFORMATION   ID number: _____   Ward: _____

Name: _____   Physician: _____

Address: _____   Date Admitted: _____

_____   Phone: _____

City: _____   State: _____   Zip: _____

Date of Birth: _____   Sex: _____   Race: _____

HEMATOLOGY

Test	Reference Ranges	Date: Time:	Date: Time:	Date: Time:	Date: Time:	Date: Time:

Hemoglobin (g/dL)
  Male
  Female
	14.0–18.0
	12.0–15.0					

Hematocrit (%)
  Male
  Female
	40–54
	35–49					

RBC ($\times 10^{12}$/L)
  Male
  Female
	4.6–6.6
	4.0–5.4					

WBC ($\times 10^{9}$/L)	4.5–11.5					
MCV (fL)	80–94					
MCHC (g/dL or %)	32–36					
MCH (pg)	26–32					
Platelet Count ($\times 10^{9}$/L)	150–450					
RDW (%)	11.5–14.5					
Reticulocyte Count						
Segmented Neutrophils (%)	50–70					
Lymphocytes (%)	18–42					
Monocytes (%)	2–11					
Basophils (%)	0–2					
Eosinophils (%)	1–3					

Erythrocyte Sed Rate (ESR)
  Male
  Female
	0–9 mm/hr
	0–15 mm/hr					

Prothrombin Time (PT)	<2-sec deviation from control; 12–14 sec					
Activated Partial Thromboplastin Time (APTT)	<35 sec					
Fibrin Degradation Products (FDP)	4.9 ± 2.8 µg FDP/mL					
Thrombin Time	15 sec					
D-Dimer	<0.5 µg/mL					

UNIVERSITY MEDICAL CENTER
CONFIDENTIAL PATIENT INFORMATION
CUMULATIVE SUMMARY REPORT

PATIENT INFORMATION   ID number: _____   Ward: _____

Name: _____   Physician: _____

Address: _____   Date Admitted: _____

_____   Phone: _____

City: _____   State: _____   Zip: _____

Date of Birth: _____   Sex: _____   Race: _____

MICROBIOLOGY

Date and Time	Procedure / Specimen	Direct Smear	Preliminary Report	Final Report

CASE SUMMARY

A. Provide a brief summary of possible patient outcomes based on the laboratory test results and the patient's diagnoses.

_____
_____
_____
_____
_____
_____
_____
_____

B. Identify the learning points that you consider helpful in working up this patient's case. *(This will be an individual response.)*

_____
_____
_____
_____
_____
_____
_____
_____
_____

NOTES

_____
_____
_____
_____
_____
_____
_____

► PATIENT'S RECORDS

PATIENT NAME: **Beatrice West**

PATIENT IDENTIFICATION NUMBER: **131425**

PHYSICIAN: **Abbey**

PATIENT INFORMATION

NAME: Beatrice West   ID NUMBER: 131425

PHYSICIAN: Abbey

DATE ADMITTED: 3/30/01   TIME: 1300

ADDRESS: 648 Shallow Grave Street, Tent City, FL 33721

PHONE: 210-555-2221

DATE OF BIRTH: 6/30/45   SEX: F   RACE: W   WARD: 2N

ADMISSION INFORMATION

WT.: 175 lb   HT.: 5'7"   B/P: 120/70

R: 18   PULSE: 86   TEMP.: 101.2

ADMISSION DIAGNOSIS

Fever of unknown origin; possible septicemia

PRIMARY COMPLAINT

Fever, malaise, abdominal pain

PATIENT HISTORY

This patient is a 55-year-old female who presented with fever, malaise, and abdominal pain. Several days prior, the patient became febrile of unknown origin. No other background history was noted at the time of admission.

TREATMENT PLAN

Radiology Ordered: Chest x-ray
Laboratory Tests Ordered: CBC, blood cultures, glucose, BUN, electrolytes

PROGRESS REPORTS

4/1/01, 1800: Bone marrow aspiration was requested based on the CBC results.

Induction chemotherapy was started.

Treatment Plan:

Laboratory Tests Ordered: Bone marrow studies. Culture for bacteria, fungi, AFB

4/5/01, 1500: Patient had a temperature spike of 101°F. The patient was disoriented, and a reddish nodular rash was noted on her trunk and extremities. Chest x-ray showed bilateral interstitial pulmonary infiltrates, and the patient was placed on a mechanical ventilator.

Antimicrobial regimen included vancomycin, ticarcillin, erythromycin, gentamicin, and amphotericin B.

Treatment Plan:

Laboratory Tests Ordered: Biopsy of lesions on trunk and extremities for bacterial culture, fungi, and AFB. Blood cultures × 3.
  Repeat CBC.

4/7/01, 0600:

Laboratory Tests Ordered: A serum latex agglutination test for cryptococcal antigen (LCAT) was requested.
  Repeat CBC.

4/13/01, 1100: The patient did not respond to the amphotericin B therapy. She became unstable, suffered cardiac arrest, and expired.

LEARNING ACTIVITIES

PATIENT: **Beatrice West**
INSTRUCTIONS: *Before you begin, read the instructions carefully and follow each step in the process.*

STUDY GUIDES

Goal A

The goal in this activity is for you to relate laboratory findings with Ms. West's symptoms on her admission to the hospital. This learning activity will allow you to collect and assess initial data pertaining to Ms. West.

Learning Issues

ISSUE 1: Identify factors in her clinical history that predispose Ms. West to her condition.

ISSUE 2: Identify the significance of this information for your attempt to determine the etiology of her condition.

Study Questions A

1. Review the patient's medical records and determine which of the presenting symptoms and which elements of the background history the physician may consider significant in her illness.

CLINICAL SYMPTOMS:

_____
_____
_____
_____

BACKGROUND HISTORY:

_____
_____
_____
_____

2. What factors predispose Ms. West to her condition, based on her clinical history?

_____
_____
_____
_____

3. In the space provided, list the laboratory tests that were requested at the time of Ms. West's admission to the facility. Which of the tests requested specifically correlate with her presenting symptoms? Highlight these tests.

4. Now access the laboratory test results from the Laboratory Information System (LIS) in the CD-ROM. Obtain Ms. West's results and record them on the patient laboratory tests results forms provided in this workbook. Review Ms. West's laboratory test results at the time she was admitted to the hospital.

    Note: If this is your first time accessing information in the CD-ROM, make sure that you start with "Before you begin."

5. a. Are any of the laboratory test results outside the usual acceptable range? If so, what do these results suggest?

    b. Based on these test results, what types of conditions would Ms. West be at risk for?

6. Are there other laboratory findings that you consider significant in this case, given the background history of the patient (e.g., culture results)?

Goal B

In this portion of the learning activity, the goal is for you to evaluate the patient's laboratory test results and determine how these results relate to her prognosis and ultimate outcome.

Learning Issues

ISSUE 1: Ascertain why the bone marrow results are significant parameters in the diagnosis of this disease.

ISSUE 2: Consider the significance of the request for a latex agglutination test for cryptococcal antigen.

Study Questions B

1. Access the LIS on the CD-ROM for the identification of the organisms isolated from the sputum and blood cultures. Use the microbiology laboratory worksheets provided in this workbook to record the microscopic findings, biochemical tests performed, appropriate results, and identification of the organism(s). What organism(s) was (were) isolated from the blood cultures and biopsy of skin lesions?

2. How do these findings correlate with Ms. West's clinical diagnosis?

3. What errors may be made in isolating and identifying this particular organism? What would be the consequences?

UNIVERSITY MEDICAL CENTER

Name: _____ Date: _____

Record #: _____ Time: _____

ANTIBODY IDENTIFICATION PANEL

Vial	Special Type	Donor	D	C	c	E	e	f	V	Cw	K	k	Kp_a	Kp_b	Js_a	Js_b	Fy_a	Fy_b	Jk_a	Jk_b	Le_a	Le_b	P1	M	N	S	s	LU_a	LU_b	Xg_a		37	AGH	CC
													Rh-Hr →|			Kell				Duffy		Kidd		Lewis		P	MN				Lutheran		Xg		Test Methods		
1	Bg(a+)	R1R1 B1080	+	+	0	0	+	0	0	0	0	+	0	+	0	+	+	0	0	+	0	+	+	+	+	+	+	0	+	+	1			
2		R1WR1 B1102	+	+	0	0	+	0	0	+	0	+	0	+	0	+	0	+	+	+	0	+	+	0	+	0	+	0	+	0	2			
3	Bg(a+)	R2R2 C1243	+	0	+	+	0	0	0	0	0	+	0	+	0	+	+	+	0	0	0	+	+	+	0	0	+	0	+	+	3			
4		ROR D575	+	0	+	0	+	+	0	0	0	+	0	+	0	+	0	0	+	+	0	0	+	+	+	0	+	0	+	0	4			
5		r'r E370	0	+	+	0	+	+	0	0	0	+	0	+	0	+	+	+	0	+	0	+	+	+	+	+	+	0	+	0	5			
6		r"r F416	0	0	+	+	+	+	0	0	0	+	0	+	0	+	0	+	+	+	+	0	0	+	+	0	+	+	+	+	6			
7		rrK G488	0	0	+	0	+	+	0	0	+	+	0	+	0	+	0	+	0	+	+	0	0	+	0	0	+	0	+	0	7			
8	Yt(b+)	rrFya H347	0	0	+	0	+	+	0	0	0	+	0	+	0	+	+	0	+	0	0	+	+	+	+	+	+	0	+	0	8			
9		rr N1434	0	0	+	0	+	+	0	0	0	+	0	+	0	+	+	+	+	+	0	0	+	+	0	+	0	0	+	+	9			
10	Co(b+)	R2R2 C199	+	0	+	+	0	0	0	0	0	+	0	+	0	+	0	+	+	0	+	0	+	+	+	0	+	0	+	+	10			
TC	He+	R1R2 A1086	+	+	+	+	+	0	0	0	0	+	0	+	0	+	0	+	0	+	0	+	+	+	+	+	+	+	+	0	TC			
		Patient's Cells																																

UNIVERSITY MEDICAL CENTER

Name: _____

Record #: _____

Date: _____

Time: _____

Cell Tests

Anti-A	_____
Anti-B	_____
Anti-D IS	_____
Anti-D 37	_____
Anti-D AHG	_____
Anti-A$_1$ Lectin	_____

Serum Tests

A$_1$ Cells	_____
A$_2$ Cells	_____
B Cells	_____

	RT	37	AHG	CC
Screen Cells I	_____	_____	_____	_____
Screen Cells II	_____	_____	_____	_____
Screen Cells III	_____	_____	_____	_____

UNIVERSITY MEDICAL CENTER
CONFIDENTIAL PATIENT INFORMATION
CUMULATIVE SUMMARY REPORT

PATIENT INFORMATION   ID number: _____   Ward: _____

Name: _____   Physician: _____

Address: _____   Date Admitted: _____

_____   Phone: _____

City: _____   State: _____   Zip: _____

Date of Birth: _____   Sex: _____   Race: _____

CHEMISTRY

Tests	Reference Ranges	Date: Time:	Date: Time:	Date: Time:	Date: Time:	Date: Time:
Acid Phos	2.5–11.7 U/L					
ACTH	9–52 pg/mL					
ALT	0–45 IU/L					
Albumin	3.5–5.0 g/dL					
A/G Ratio	0.7–2.1					
Aldosterone	??					
Alkaline Phos	41–137 IU/L					
Ammonia	11–35 µmol/L					
Amylase	95–290 U/L					
Anion Gap	10–18 mmol/L					
AST	0–41 IU/L					
Bilirubin	0.2–1.0 mg/dL					
Bilirubin (direct)	0.2–1.0 mg/dL					
BUN	10–20 mg/dL					
Calcium (total)	4.3–5.3 mEq/L					
Calcuim (ionized)	1.16–1.32 mmol/L					
Chloride	95–100 mmol/L					
Carbon Dioxide	23–32 mmol/L					

CHEMISTRY (page 2)

Tests	Reference Ranges	Date: Time:	Date: Time:	Date: Time:	Date: Time:	Date: Time:
Cholesterol	<200 mg/dL					
CK	15–160 U/L					
CK-MB	15–160 U/L					
Creatinine	0.7–1.5 mg/dL					
Creatintine Clearance	80–120 mL/min					
GGT	6–45 U/L					
Globulin	2.3–3.2 g/dL					
Glucose	65–105 mg/dL					
LD	100–225 U/L					
LDL Cholesterol	75–140 U/L					
LDL/HDL	2.9–2.2					
Lipase	0–1.0 U/mL					
Magnesium	1.3–2.1 mEq/L					
Osmolality	275–295 mOsM/kg					
Phosphorus	2.7–4.5 mg/dL					
Potassium	3.5–5.0 mmol/L					
Protein	5.8–8.2 g/dL					
Sodium	135–145 mmol/L					
Triglycerides	10–190 mg/dL					
Uric Acid	3.5–7.2 mg/dL					
HCO_3	100–225 U/L					

UNIVERSITY MEDICAL CENTER
CONFIDENTIAL PATIENT INFORMATION
CUMULATIVE SUMMARY REPORT

PATIENT INFORMATION   ID number: _____   Ward: _____

Name: _____   Physician: _____

Address: _____   Date Admitted: _____

_____   Phone: _____

City: _____   State: _____   Zip: _____

Date of Birth: _____   Sex: _____   Race: _____

HEMATOLOGY

Test	Reference Ranges	Date: Time:	Date: Time:	Date: Time:	Date: Time:	Date: Time:
Hemoglobin (g/dL) Male Female	14.0–18.0 12.0–15.0					
Hematocrit (%) Male Female	40–54 35–49					
RBC ($\times 10^{12}$/L) Male Female	4.6–6.6 4.0–5.4					
WBC ($\times 10^9$/L)	4.5–11.5					
MCV (fL)	80–94					
MCHC (g/dL or %)	32–36					
MCH (pg)	26–32					
Platelet Count ($\times 10^9$/L)	150–450					
RDW (%)	11.5–14.5					
Reticulocyte Count						
Segmented Neutrophils (%)	50–70					
Lymphocytes (%)	18–42					
Monocytes (%)	2–11					
Basophils (%)	0–2					
Eosinophils (%)	1–3					
Erythrocyte Sed Rate (ESR) Male Female	0–9 mm/hr 0–15 mm/hr					
Prothrombin Time (PT)	<2-sec deviation from control; 12–14 sec					
Activated Partial Thromboplastin Time (APTT)	<35 sec					
Fibrin Degradation Products (FDP)	4.9 ± 2.8 µg FDP/mL					
Thrombin Time	15 sec					
D-Dimer	<0.5 µg/mL					

UNIVERSITY MEDICAL CENTER
CONFIDENTIAL PATIENT INFORMATION
CUMULATIVE SUMMARY REPORT

PATIENT INFORMATION   ID number: _____   Ward: _____

Name: _____   Physician: _____

Address: _____   Date Admitted: _____

_____   Phone: _____

City: _____   State: _____   Zip: _____

Date of Birth: _____   Sex: _____   Race: _____

MICROBIOLOGY

Date and Time	Procedure / Specimen	Direct Smear	Preliminary Report	Final Report

CASE SUMMARY

A. Provide a brief summary of possible patient outcomes based on the laboratory test results and the patient's diagnoses.

B. Identify the learning points that you consider helpful in working up this patient's case. *(This will be an individual response.)*

NOTES

▶ PATIENT'S RECORDS

PATIENT NAME: **Lena Wilson**

PATIENT IDENTIFICATION NUMBER: **567123**

PHYSICIAN: **Craig**

PATIENT INFORMATION

NAME: Lena Wilson   ID NUMBER: 567123

PHYSICIAN: Craig

DATE ADMITTED: 6/11/02   TIME: 1300

ADDRESS: 5020 Seyne St., Looney, ND 80983

PHONE: 221-111-2222

DATE OF BIRTH: 2/13/64   SEX: F   RACE: W   WARD: 4W

ADMISSION INFORMATION

WT.: 100 lb   HT.: 4'6"   B/P: 102/68

R: 18   PULSE: 100   TEMP.: 101.6

ADMISSION DIAGNOSIS
Anemia, thrombocytopenia

PRIMARY COMPLAINT
Shortness of breath, chest pain, pain in muscles of upper back, fatigue after climbing one flight of stairs or walking 100 m

PATIENT HISTORY

A 38-year-old Caucasian female presented with symptoms of new-onset shortness of breath for the past 2 days, chest pain in the muscles of the upper back, fatigue after climbing one flight of stairs or walking 100 m, and no evidence of gross blood loss to explain these symptoms. The patient was diagnosed with AML M4 15 months prior. Treatment included chemotherapeutic drugs and a bone marrow transplant. A bone marrow biopsy 10 months prior to this visit indicated complete remission.

TREATMENT PLAN

Laboratory Tests Ordered: CBC. Type and cross-match for 2 units of packed RBCs. Total bilirubin.

PROGRESS REPORTS

6/12/02, 1800: The patient was given 6 units of platelets and 2 units of packed RBCs. The patient became stabilized.

Treatment Plan: Evaluate lab results. Request bone marrow aspiration and flow cytometry studies.

6/17/02, 0600: The patient remained stable. The patient was placed on chemotherapy.

Treatment Plan: Hemoglobin, hematocrit, platelet count daily.

6/20/02, 0900: Discharge patient. Follow up in outpatient clinic.

LEARNING ACTIVITIES

PATIENT: Lena Wilson
INSTRUCTIONS: *Before you begin, read the instructions carefully and follow each step in the process.*

STUDY GUIDES

Goal A

The goal in this activity is for you to relate laboratory findings with Ms. Wilson's symptoms on her admission to the hospital. This learning activity will allow you to collect and assess initial data pertaining to Ms. Wilson.

Learning Issues

ISSUE 1: Identify clinical symptoms that indicate Ms. Wilson's condition based on her history.

ISSUE 2: Determine why immunologic marker results are significant parameters in monitoring this disease process.

ISSUE 3: Determine how the differential diagnosis is made based on cellular morphologic features and flow cytometry studies.

Study Questions A

1. Review the patient's medical records and determine which of the presenting symptoms and which elements of the background history the physician may consider significant in her illness.

CLINICAL SYMPTOMS:

_____

_____

_____

_____

BACKGROUND HISTORY:

_____

_____

_____

2. In the space provided, list the laboratory tests that were requested at the time of Ms. Wilson's admission to the facility. Which of the tests specifically requested correlate with her presenting symptoms? Highlight these tests.

_____

_____

_____

_____

3. Now access the laboratory test results from the Laboratory Information System (LIS) in the CD-ROM. Obtain Ms. Wilson's results and record them on the patient laboratory tests results forms provided in this workbook. Review Ms. Wilson's laboratory test results at the time she was admitted to the hospital.

    Note: If this is your first time accessing information in the CD-ROM, make sure that you start with "Before you begin."

4. a. Are any of the laboratory test results outside the usual acceptable range? If so, what do these results suggest?

    _____

    _____

    _____

    _____

    b. How do these tests result correlate with Ms. Wilson's presenting symptoms?

    _____

    _____

    _____

    _____

5. Are there other laboratory findings that you consider significant in this case, given the background history of the patient?

    _____

    _____

    _____

    _____

Goal B

In this portion of the learning activity, the goal is for you to evaluate the patient's laboratory test results and determine how these results relate to her prognosis and ultimate outcome.

Learning Issues

ISSUE 1: Determine how a differential diagnosis is made based on cellular morphologic features and flow cytometry studies.

ISSUE 2: Evaluate the use of the labarotory in this case.

Study Questions B

1. a. Which of the laboratory test results support, confirm, or reject the initial diagnosis?

    _____

    _____

    _____

   b. Review the peripheral blood smear results. Access the LIS on the CD-ROM to obtain the hematology findings. What morphologic characteristics led to the diagnosis of this patient's condition?

    _____

    _____

    _____

    _____

   c. How is the investigation carried out to confirm the diagnosis?

    _____

    _____

    _____

    _____

2. How do cell surface markers differentiate this disease condition from others?

    _____

    _____

    _____

    _____

3. Is the laboratory appropriately used? Support your answer. *(This will be an individual response.)*

    _____

    _____

    _____

    _____

UNIVERSITY MEDICAL CENTER

Name: _____

Record #: _____

Date: _____

Time: _____

ANTIBODY IDENTIFICATION PANEL

Vial	Special Type	Donor	D	C	c	E	e	f	V	Cw	K	k	Kpa	Kpb	Jsa	Jsb	Fya	Fyb	Jka	Jkb	Lea	Leb	P1	M	N	S	s	LUa	LUb	Xga	37	AGH	CC
						Rh-Hr								Kell				Duffy		Kidd		Lewis		P		MN				Lutheran		Xg		Test Methods	
1	Bg(a+)	R1R1 B1080	+	+	0	0	+	0	0	0	0	+	0	+	0	+	+	0	0	+	0	+	+	+	+	+	+	0	+	+	1		
2		R1WR1 B1102	+	+	0	0	+	0	0	+	+	+	0	+	0	+	0	+	+	+	0	+	+	0	+	0	+	0	+	0	2		
3	Bg(a+)	R2R2 C1243	+	0	+	+	0	0	0	0	0	+	0	+	0	+	+	0	0	+	0	+	+	+	0	+	+	0	+	+	3		
4		ROR D575	+	0	+	0	+	+	0	0	0	+	0	+	0	+	0	0	+	0	0	0	+	0	+	0	+	0	+	+	4		
5		r'r E370	0	+	+	0	+	+	0	0	0	+	0	+	0	+	+	+	+	+	0	+	+	+	+	+	+	0	+	0	5		
6		r"r F416	0	0	+	+	+	+	0	0	0	+	0	+	0	+	+	+	+	+	+	+	0	+	+	0	+	+	+	+	6		
7		rrK G488	0	0	+	0	+	+	0	0	+	+	0	+	0	+	0	+	+	0	+	0	0	+	0	0	+	0	+	0	7		
8	Yt(b+)	rrFya H347	0	0	+	0	+	+	0	0	0	+	0	+	0	+	+	0	+	+	0	0	+	+	+	+	+	0	+	0	8		
9		rr N1434	0	0	+	0	+	+	0	0	0	+	0	+	0	+	+	+	0	+	+	0	+	+	0	0	0	0	+	+	9		
10	Co(b+)	R2R2 C199	+	0	+	+	0	0	0	0	0	+	0	+	0	+	+	+	+	0	0	0	+	+	+	+	+	0	+	+	10		
TC	He+	R1R2 A1086	+	+	+	+	+	+	0	0	0	+	0	+	0	+	+	+	0	0	0	+	+	+	+	+	+	+	+	0	TC		
		Patient's Cells																															

Name: _____

Record #: _____

Date: _____

Time: _____

Cell Tests

Anti-A _____

Anti-B _____

Anti-D IS _____

Anti-D 37 _____

Anti-D AHG _____

Anti-A$_1$ Lectin _____

Serum Tests

	RT	37	AHG	CC
A$_1$ Cells	_____			
A$_2$ Cells	_____			
B Cells	_____			
Screen Cells I	_____	_____	_____	_____
Screen Cells II	_____	_____	_____	_____
Screen Cells III	_____	_____	_____	_____

UNIVERSITY MEDICAL CENTER
CONFIDENTIAL PATIENT INFORMATION
CUMULATIVE SUMMARY REPORT

PATIENT INFORMATION   ID number: _____   Ward: _____

Name: _____   Physician: _____

Address: _____   Date Admitted: _____

_____   Phone: _____

City: _____   State: _____   Zip: _____

Date of Birth: _____   Sex: _____   Race: _____

CHEMISTRY

Tests	Reference Ranges	Date: Time:	Date: Time:	Date: Time:	Date: Time:	Date: Time:
Acid Phos	2.5–11.7 U/L					
ACTH	9–52 pg/mL					
ALT	0–45 IU/L					
Albumin	3.5–5.0 g/dL					
A/G Ratio	0.7–2.1					
Aldosterone	??					
Alkaline Phos	41–137 IU/L					
Ammonia	11–35 µmol/L					
Amylase	95–290 U/L					
Anion Gap	10–18 mmol/L					
AST	0–41 IU/L					
Bilirubin	0.2–1.0 mg/dL					
Bilirubin (direct)	0.2–1.0 mg/dL					
BUN	10–20 mg/dL					
Calcium (total)	4.3–5.3 mEq/L					
Calcuim (ionized)	1.16–1.32 mmol/L					
Chloride	95–100 mmol/L					
Carbon Dioxide	23–32 mmol/L					

CHEMISTRY (page 2)

Tests	Reference Ranges	Date: Time:	Date: Time:	Date: Time:	Date: Time:	Date: Time:
Cholesterol	<200 mg/dL					
CK	15–160 U/L					
CK-MB	15–160 U/L					
Creatinine	0.7–1.5 mg/dL					
Creatintine Clearance	80–120 mL/min					
GGT	6–45 U/L					
Globulin	2.3–3.2 g/dL					
Glucose	65–105 mg/dL					
LD	100–225 U/L					
LDL Cholesterol	75–140 U/L					
LDL/HDL	2.9–2.2					
Lipase	0–1.0 U/mL					
Magnesium	1.3–2.1 mEq/L					
Osmolality	275–295 mOsM/kg					
Phosphorus	2.7–4.5 mg/dL					
Potassium	3.5–5.0 mmol/L					
Protein	5.8–8.2 g/dL					
Sodium	135–145 mmol/L					
Triglycerides	10–190 mg/dL					
Uric Acid	3.5–7.2 mg/dL					
HCO_3	100–225 U/L					

PATIENT INFORMATION   ID number: _____   Ward: _____

Name: _____   Physician: _____

Address: _____   Date Admitted: _____

_____   Phone: _____

City: _____   State: _____   Zip: _____

Date of Birth: _____   Sex: _____   Race: _____

HEMATOLOGY

Test	Reference Ranges	Date: Time:	Date: Time:	Date: Time:	Date: Time:	Date: Time:
Hemoglobin (g/dL) Male Female	14.0–18.0 12.0–15.0					
Hematocrit (%) Male Female	40–54 35–49					
RBC ($\times 10^{12}$/L) Male Female	4.6–6.6 4.0–5.4					
WBC ($\times 10^{9}$/L)	4.5–11.5					
MCV (fL)	80–94					
MCHC (g/dL or %)	32–36					
MCH (pg)	26–32					
Platelet Count ($\times 10^{9}$/L)	150–450					
RDW (%)	11.5–14.5					
Reticulocyte Count						
Segmented Neutrophils (%)	50–70					
Lymphocytes (%)	18–42					
Monocytes (%)	2–11					
Basophils (%)	0–2					
Eosinophils (%)	1–3					
Erythrocyte Sed Rate (ESR) Male Female	0–9 mm/hr 0–15 mm/hr					
Prothrombin Time (PT)	<2-sec deviation from control; 12–14 sec					
Activated Partial Thromboplastin Time (APTT)	<35 sec					
Fibrin Degradation Products (FDP)	4.9 ± 2.8 µg FDP/mL					
Thrombin Time	15 sec					
D-Dimer	<0.5 µg/mL					

UNIVERSITY MEDICAL CENTER
CONFIDENTIAL PATIENT INFORMATION
CUMULATIVE SUMMARY REPORT

PATIENT INFORMATION   ID number: _____   Ward: _____

Name: _____   Physician: _____

Address: _____   Date Admitted: _____

_____   Phone: _____

City: _____   State: _____   Zip: _____

Date of Birth: _____   Sex: _____   Race: _____

MICROBIOLOGY				
Date and Time	**Procedure / Specimen**	**Direct Smear**	**Preliminary Report**	**Final Report**

CASE SUMMARY

A. Provide a brief summary of possible patient outcomes based on the laboratory test results and the patient's diagnoses.

_____

_____

_____

_____

_____

_____

_____

_____

B. Identify the learning points that you consider helpful in working up this patient's case. *(This will be an individual response.)*

_____

_____

_____

_____

_____

_____

_____

_____

_____

NOTES

_____

_____

_____

_____

_____

_____

_____

► PATIENT'S RECORDS

PATIENT NAME: **Dannon Wise**

PATIENT IDENTIFICATION NUMBER: **102248**

PHYSICIAN: **Lipton**

PATIENT INFORMATION

NAME: Dannon Wise   ID NUMBER: 102248

PHYSICIAN: Lipton

DATE ADMITTED: 1/2/00   TIME: 1300

ADDRESS: 5900 Benita Ave., Washington, DC 20202

PHONE: 202 555-1234

DATE OF BIRTH: 5/11/20   SEX: F   RACE: B   WARD: 3N

ADMISSION INFORMATION

WT.: 120 lb   HT.: 5'3"   B/P: 110/70

R: 22   PULSE: 80   TEMP.: 102

ANTIBIOTICS TAKEN:

ADMISSION DIAGNOSIS
Pneumonia

PRIMARY COMPLAINT
Fever, lack of appetite, dehydration, lethargy

PATIENT HISTORY

The patient is an 79-year-old female who was admitted from the nursing home. At the time of admission, the patient was febrile and confused, and seemed lethargic. The nursing home staff reported that the patient refused to eat and drink. Past history included osteomyelitis of the foot, renal disease, heart failure, diverticulitis, and diabetes. The patient also had a history of alcohol abuse and heavy smoking.

TREATMENT PLAN

Radiology Ordered: Chest x-ray
Laboratory Tests Ordered: Glucose, BUN, electrolytes, urinalysis, CBC

PROGRESS REPORTS

1/2/00: Chest x-ray clear. Patient remained febrile and confused.

Treatment Plan: Performed lumbar puncture to obtain cerebrospinal fluid. Collected blood cultures × 3 every 30 min.

1/2/00, 2300: The patient was placed on ampicillin and penicillin. Later, gentamicin was added to the regimen.

1/3/00, 0600: Blood cultures and CSF produced similar results. The infection was resolved uneventfully, and the patient returned to the nursing home, where she continued her treatment.

LEARNING ACTIVITIES

PATIENT: Dannon Wise
INSTRUCTIONS: *Before you begin, read the instructions carefully and follow each step in the process.*

STUDY GUIDES

Goal A

The goal in this activity is for you to relate laboratory data with Ms. Wise's previous medical history and her current clinical condition when she was transferred from the nursing home. This learning activity will allow you to collect and assess initial data pertaining to Ms. Wise.

Learning Issues

ISSUE 1: Identify risk factors in her medical history that may have predisposed Ms. Wise to her condition.

Issue 2: Identify the significance of this information for your attempt to recover the etiologic agent of her infection.

Study Questions A

1. Review the patient's medical records and determine which of the presenting symptoms and which elements of the background history the physician may consider significant in her illness.

CLINICAL SYMPTOMS:

_____

_____

_____

_____

BACKGROUND HISTORY:

_____

_____

_____

_____

2. In the space provided, list the laboratory tests that were requested at the time of Ms. Wise's admission to the facility. Which of the tests requested specifically correlate with her presenting symptoms? Highlight these tests.

_____

_____

_____

_____

3. Now access the laboratory test results from the Laboratory Information System (LIS) in the CD-ROM. Obtain Ms. Wise's results and record them on the patient laboratory tests results forms provided in this workbook. Review Ms. Wise's laboratory test results at the time she was admitted to the hospital.

   Note: If this is your first time accessing information in the CD-ROM, make sure that you start with "Before you begin."

4. Are any chemistry or hematology results outside the normal acceptable range? If so, what do these results suggest?

_____

_____

_____

_____

5. Are there other laboratory results that are relevant to this case that you need to consider?

_____

_____

_____

_____

Goal B

In this portion of the learning activity, the goal is for you to correlate the organism isolated from Ms. Wise's CSF and blood cultures with her clinical history, clinical progress, and possible outcomes of her infection.

Learning Issues

ISSUE 1: Identify the epidemiologic features associated with the organism isolated.

ISSUE 2: Differentiate the clinical and laboratory features of Ms. Wise's infection from those caused by other bacterial agents.

Study Questions B

1. Access the LIS on the CD-ROM for the identification of the organism isolated from the exudates and blood cultures. Use the microbiology laboratory worksheets provided in this workbook to record the microscopic findings, biochemical tests performed, appropriate results, and identification of the organism(s). What organism(s) was (were) isolated from the CSF and blood cultures?

_____

_____

_____

_____

2. How is this organism usually acquired?

    _____

    _____

    _____

    _____

3. Why is this patient at risk of infection with this organism?

    _____

    _____

    _____

    _____

4. What errors may be made in the clinical and laboratory diagnosis of
    this infection?

    _____

    _____

    _____

    _____

UNIVERSITY MEDICAL CENTER

Name: _____

Record #: _____

Date: _____

Time: _____

ANTIBODY IDENTIFICATION PANEL

Vial	Special Type	Donor	Rh-Hr								Kell						Duffy		Kidd		Lewis		P	MN				Lutheran		Xg	Test Methods			
			D	C	c	E	e	f	V	Cw	K	k	Kp$_a$	Kp$_b$	Js$_a$	Js$_b$	Fy$_a$	Fy$_b$	Jk$_a$	Jk$_b$	Le$_a$	Le$_b$	P1	M	N	S	s	LU$_a$	LU$_b$	Xg$_a$	37	AGH	CC	
1	Bg(a+)	R1R1 B1080	+	+	0	0	+	0	0	0	0	+	0	+	0	+	+	0	0	+	0	+	+	+	+	+	+	0	+	+				1
2		R1WR1 B1102	+	+	0	0	+	0	0	+	+	+	0	+	0	+	0	+	+	+	0	+	+	0	+	0	+	0	+	0				2
3	Bg(a+)	R2R2 C1243	+	0	+	+	0	0	0	0	0	+	0	+	0	+	+	+	0	+	0	0	+	+	0	+	+	0	+	+				3
4		ROR D575	+	0	+	0	+	+	0	0	0	+	0	+	0	+	0	0	+	0	0	0	+	0	+	0	+	0	+	+				4
5		r'r E370	0	+	+	0	+	+	0	0	0	+	0	+	0	+	+	+	0	+	0	+	+	+	+	+	+	0	+	0				5
6		r"r F416	0	0	+	+	+	+	0	0	0	+	0	+	0	+	+	+	+	+	0	+	0	+	+	0	+	+	+	+				6
7		rrK G488	0	0	+	0	+	+	0	0	+	0	0	+	0	+	0	+	0	+	+	0	0	+	0	0	+	0	+	0				7
8	Yt(b+)	rrFya H347	0	0	+	0	+	+	0	0	0	+	0	+	0	+	0	0	0	0	+	0	+	+	+	+	+	0	+	0				8
9		rr N1434	0	0	+	0	+	+	0	0	0	+	0	+	0	+	+	+	+	0	0	+	+	0	0	+	0	0	+	+				9
10	Co(b+)	R2R2 C199	+	0	+	+	0	0	0	0	0	+	0	+	0	+	0	+	+	0	+	0	0	+	+	0	+	0	+	+				10
TC	He+	R1R2 A1086	+	+	+	+	+	0	0	0	0	+	0	+	0	+	0	+	0	+	0	+	+	+	+	+	+	+	+	0				TC
		Patient's Cells																																

Name: _____

Record #: _____

Date: _____

Time: _____

Cell Tests

Anti-A _____

Anti-B _____

Anti-D IS _____

Anti-D 37 _____

Anti-D AHG _____

Anti-A$_1$ Lectin _____

Serum Tests

	RT	37	AHG	CC
A$_1$ Cells	_____			
A$_2$ Cells	_____			
B Cells	_____			
Screen Cells I	_____	_____	_____	_____
Screen Cells II	_____	_____	_____	_____
Screen Cells III	_____	_____	_____	_____

357

UNIVERSITY MEDICAL CENTER
CONFIDENTIAL PATIENT INFORMATION
CUMULATIVE SUMMARY REPORT

PATIENT INFORMATION   ID number: _____   Ward: _____

Name: _____   Physician: _____

Address: _____   Date Admitted: _____

_____   Phone: _____

City: _____   State: _____   Zip: _____

Date of Birth: _____   Sex: _____   Race: _____

CHEMISTRY

Tests	Reference Ranges	Date: Time:	Date: Time:	Date: Time:	Date: Time:	Date: Time:
Acid Phos	2.5–11.7 U/L					
ACTH	9–52 pg/mL					
ALT	0–45 IU/L					
Albumin	3.5–5.0 g/dL					
A/G Ratio	0.7–2.1					
Aldosterone	??					
Alkaline Phos	41–137 IU/L					
Ammonia	11–35 μmol/L					
Amylase	95–290 U/L					
Anion Gap	10–18 mmol/L					
AST	0–41 IU/L					
Bilirubin	0.2–1.0 mg/dL					
Bilirubin (direct)	0.2–1.0 mg/dL					
BUN	10–20 mg/dL					
Calcium (total)	4.3–5.3 mEq/L					
Calcuim (ionized)	1.16–1.32 mmol/L					
Chloride	95–100 mmol/L					
Carbon Dioxide	23–32 mmol/L					

CHEMISTRY (page 2)

Tests	Reference Ranges	Date: Time:	Date: Time:	Date: Time:	Date: Time:	Date: Time:
Cholesterol	<200 mg/dL					
CK	15–160 U/L					
CK-MB	15–160 U/L					
Creatinine	0.7–1.5 mg/dL					
Creatintine Clearance	80–120 mL/min					
GGT	6–45 U/L					
Globulin	2.3–3.2 g/dL					
Glucose	65–105 mg/dL					
LD	100–225 U/L					
LDL Cholesterol	75–140 U/L					
LDL/HDL	2.9–2.2					
Lipase	0–1.0 U/mL					
Magnesium	1.3–2.1 mEq/L					
Osmolality	275–295 mOsM/kg					
Phosphorus	2.7–4.5 mg/dL					
Potassium	3.5–5.0 mmol/L					
Protein	5.8–8.2 g/dL					
Sodium	135–145 mmol/L					
Triglycerides	10–190 mg/dL					
Uric Acid	3.5–7.2 mg/dL					
HCO_3	100–225 U/L					

UNIVERSITY MEDICAL CENTER
CONFIDENTIAL PATIENT INFORMATION
CUMULATIVE SUMMARY REPORT

PATIENT INFORMATION   ID number: _____   Ward: _____

Name: _____   Physician: _____

Address: _____   Date Admitted: _____

_____   Phone: _____

City: _____   State: _____   Zip: _____

Date of Birth: _____   Sex: _____   Race: _____

HEMATOLOGY

Test	Reference Ranges	Date: Time:	Date: Time:	Date: Time:	Date: Time:	Date: Time:
Hemoglobin (g/dL) Male Female	14.0–18.0 12.0–15.0					
Hematocrit (%) Male Female	40–54 35–49					
RBC ($\times 10^{12}$/L) Male Female	4.6–6.6 4.0–5.4					
WBC ($\times 10^{9}$/L)	4.5–11.5					
MCV (fL)	80–94					
MCHC (g/dL or %)	32–36					
MCH (pg)	26–32					
Platelet Count ($\times 10^{9}$/L)	150–450					
RDW (%)	11.5–14.5					
Reticulocyte Count						
Segmented Neutrophils (%)	50–70					
Lymphocytes (%)	18–42					
Monocytes (%)	2–11					
Basophils (%)	0–2					
Eosinophils (%)	1–3					
Erythrocyte Sed Rate (ESR) Male Female	0–9 mm/hr 0–15 mm/hr					
Prothrombin Time (PT)	<2-sec deviation from control; 12–14 sec					
Activated Partial Thromboplastin Time (APTT)	<35 sec					
Fibrin Degradation Products (FDP)	4.9 ± 2.8 µg FDP/mL					
Thrombin Time	15 sec					
D-Dimer	<0.5 µg/mL					

PATIENT INFORMATION   ID number: _____   Ward: _____

Name: _____   Physician: _____

Address: _____   Date Admitted: _____

_____   Phone: _____

City: _____   State: _____   Zip: _____

Date of Birth: _____   Sex: _____   Race: _____

MICROBIOLOGY

Date and Time	Procedure / Specimen	Direct Smear	Preliminary Report	Final Report

CASE SUMMARY

A. Provide a brief summary of possible patient outcomes based on the laboratory test results and the patient's diagnoses.

B. Identify the learning points that you consider helpful in working up this patient's case. *(This will be an individual response.)*

NOTES

▶ APPENDIX A

ANTIGENS

Antigen System	Antigen Name	ISBT Number	Antigen Freq. % W	B	RBC Antigen Expression at Birth	Antigen Distrib. Plasma/RBC	Demonstrates Dosage	Antigen Modification Enzyme/Other
Rh	D	RH1	85	92	strong	RBC only	no	Enz. ↑
	C	RH2	70	34	strong	RBC only	yes	Enz. ↑
	E	RH3	30	21	strong	RBC only	yes	Enz. ↑
	c	RH4	80	97	strong	RBC only	yes	Enz. ↑
	e	RH5	98	99	strong	RBC only	yes	Enz. ↑
	ce/f	RH6	64		strong	RBC only	no	Enz. ↑
	Ce	RH7	70		strong	RBC only	no	Enz. ↑
	C^w	RH8	1	rare	strong	RBC only	yes	Enz. ↑
	G	RH12	86		strong	RBC only	no	Enz. ↑
	V	RH10	1		strong	RBC only	no	Enz. ↑
	VS	RH20	1		strong	RBC only	no	
Kell	K	K1	9	rare	strong	RBC only	occ	Enz. → AET+ ↓ ZZAP ↓ ++
	k	K2	98.8	100	strong	RBC only	occ	Enz. → AET+ ↓ ZZAP ↓ ++
	Kp^a	K3	2	rare	strong	RBC only	occ	Enz. → AET+ ↓ ZZAP ↓ ++
	Kp^b	K4	99.9	100	strong	RBC only	occ	Enz. → AET+ ↓ ZZAP ↓ ++
	Js^a	K6	1	20	strong	RBC only	occ	Enz. → AET+ ↓ ZZAP ↓ ++
	Js^b	K7	99.9	99	strong	RBC only	occ	Enz. → AET+ ↓ ZZAP ↓ ++
	Kx	—	99.9	99.9	weak	RBC low	occ	Enz. → AET+ ↑ ZZAP ↑ ++
Duffy	Fy^a	FY1	65	10	strong	RBC only	yes	Enz. ↓ AET ↓ ZZAP ↓
	Fy^b	FY2	80	23	strong	RBC only	yes	Enz ↓ AET ↓ ZZAP ↓
		FY3	100		strong	RBC only	no	Enz. → AET ↓ ZZAP ↓
		FY4	5	rare	strong	RBC only	?	Enz. → AET ↓
		FY5	100		?	?	no	Enz. → AET ↓ ZZAP ↓
		FY6	100	?	?	RBC only	?	Enz. ↓ AET → ZZAP ↓

*It has been found that Kx is inherited independently of the Kell system; consequently it is no longer referred to as K15.

Abbreviations: AET = 2-aminoetylisothiouronium; ↑ enhanced reactivity; → no effect; HDN = hemolytic disease of the newborn; HTR = hemolytic transfusion reaction; NRBC = non-red blood cell; RBC = red blood cell; WBC = white blood cell; ZZAP = dithiothreitol plus papain; ↓ depressed reactivity.

ANTIBODIES

Stimulation	Serology Saline	AHG	Comp. Binding	Immunogloblin Class IgM	IgG	Optimum Temperature	Clinical Significance HTR	HDN	Comments
RBC	occ	yes	no	occ	yes	warm	yes	yes	Very rarely IgA anti-D may be produced; however, this is invariable with IgG.
RBC	occ	yes	no	occ	yes	warm	yes	yes	
RBC/NRBC	occ	yes	no	occ	yes	warm	yes	yes	Anti-E may often occur without obvious immune stimulation.
RBC	occ	yes	no	occ	yes	warm	yes	yes	
RBC	occ	yes	no	occ	yes	warm	yes	yes	Warm autoantibodies often appear to have anti-e-like specificity.
RBC	occ	yes	no	occ	yes	warm	yes	?	
RBC	occ	yes	no	occ	yes	warm	yes	yes	
RBC/NRBC	occ	yes	no	occ	yes	warm	yes	yes	Anti-C^W may often occur without obvious immune stimulation.
RBC	occ	yes	no	occ	yes	warm	yes	yes	
RBC	occ	yes	no	occ	yes	warm	yes	yes	Antibodies to V and VS present problems only in the black population, where the antigen frequencies are in the order of 20 to 25.
RBC	occ	yes	no	occ	yes	warm	yes	yes	
RBC	occ	yes	some	occ	yes	warm	yes	yes	Some antibodies to Kell system have been reported to react poorly in low ionic media.
RBC	no	yes	no	no	yes	warm	yes	yes	
RBC	no	yes	no	no	yes	warm	yes	yes	Kell system antigens are destroyed by AET and by ZZAP.
RBC	no	yes	no	no	yes	warm	yes	yes	
RBC	no	yes	no	no	yes	warm	yes	yes	Anti-K1 has been reported to occur following bacterial infection.
RBC	no	yes	no	no	yes	warm	yes	yes	
RBC	no	yes	no	occ	yes	warm	yes	yes	The lack of a Kx expression on RBCs and WBCs has been associated with the McLeod phenotype and CGD.
RBC	rare	yes	some	rare	yes	warm	yes	yes	Fy(a and b) antigens are destroyed by enzymes. Fy(a$^-$ b$^-$) cells are resistant to invasion by *P. vivax* merozoites, a malaria-causing parasite.
RBC	rare	yes	some	rare	yes	warm	yes		
RBC	no	yes	?	no	yes	warm	?	yes	FY3, 4, and 5 are not destroyed by enzymes.
RBC	no	yes	some	no	yes	warm			
RBC	no	yes	?	no	yes	warm			FY5 may be formed by interaction of Rh and Duffy gene products.
RBC	no	yes	?	?	yes	warm	?	?	FY6 antibody reacts with most human red cells except Fy(a$^-$ b$^-$) and is responsible for susceptibility of cells to penetration by *P. vivax*.

ANTIGENS

Antigen System	Antigen Name	ISBT Number	Antigen Freq. % W	Antigen Freq. % B	RBC Antigen Expression at Birth	Antigen Distrib. Plasma/RBC	Demonstrates Dosage	Antigen Modification Enzyme/Other
	Jk^a	JK1	77	91	strong	RBC only	yes	Enz. ↑
Kidd	Jk^b	JK2	73	43	strong	RBC only	yes	Enz. ↑
		JK3	100	100	strong	RBC	no	Enz. ↑
Lewis	Le^a	LE1	22	23	nil	Plasma/RBC	no	Enz. ↑
	Le^b	LE2	72	55	nil	Plasma/RBC	no	Enz. ↑
P*	P$_1$	P1	79	94	moderate	RBC, platelets, WBC	individual variation	Enz. ↑ AET → ZZAP ↑
	P	P	100	100	moderate	RBC platelets, WBC	no	Enz. ↑ AET → ZZAP ↑
	p^{k**}		100	100	?	RBC, platelets, fibroblast	no	no
MNS	M	MNS1	78	70	strong	RBC only	yes	Enz. ↓ AET → ZZAP ↓
	N	MNS2	72	74	strong	RBC only	yes	Enz. ↓ AET → ZZAP ↓
	S	MNS3	55	37	strong	RBC only	yes	Enz. ↓ AET → ZZAP ↓
	s	MNS4	89	97	strong	RBC only	yes	Enz. ↓ AET → ZZAP ↓
	U	MNS5	100	100	strong	RBC only	no	Enz. → AET → ZZAP ↓
Lutheran	Lu^a	LU1	7.6	5.3	poor	RBC only	yes	Enz. → AET → ZZAP ↓
	Lu^b	LU2	99.8	99.9	poor	RBC only	yes	?
		LU3	>99.8					

*In the P system, phenotype P contains both P$_1$ and P antigens; phenotype P$_2$ contains only P antigens; phenotype p lacks both P$_1$ and P antigens.

**The p^k antigen is typically converted to P; therefore there is no p^k antigen detectable on adult cells. There are rare individuals (p$_1$^{k},p$_2$^{k}) where pk antigen is not converted to P.

Abbreviations: AET = 2-aminoethylisothiouronium; ↑ enhanced reactivity; → no effect; HDN = hemolytic disease of the newborn; HTR = hemolytic transfusion reaction; NRBC = non-red blood cell; RBC = red blood cell; WBC = white blood cell; ZZAP = dithiothreitol plus papain; ↓ depressed reactivity.

Reprinted with permission from Harmenings D: *Modern Blood Banking and Transfusion Practices*, 4th ed. Philadelphia: FA Davis, 1999.

ANTIBODIES

Stimulation	Serology: Saline	Serology: AHG	Comp. Binding	Immunoglobin Class: IgM	Immunoglobin Class: IgG	Optimum Temperature	Clinical Significance: HTR	Clinical Significance: HDN	Comments
RBC	no	yes	yes	no	yes	warm	yes	yes	Kidd antibodies seem to disappear rapidly both in vivo and in vitro. They are often associated with delayed HTR.
RBC	no	yes	yes	no	yes	warm	yes	yes	Jk(a−b−) RBCs are resistant to lysis by 2M urea.
RBC	rare	yes	?	no	yes	warm	yes	yes	
NRBC	yes	some	yes	yes	occ	cold	rare	no	Sometimes a pattern of unusual agglutination sheeting occurs.
NRBC	yes	some	yes	yes	no	cold	no	no	Antigen expression may be lost during pregnancy for Lewis system.
NRBC	yes	no	some	yes	rare	cold	yes	no	Commonly occurring antibody in P_2
NRBC	yes	occ	some	most	few	cold	yes	rare	Anti-P may occur "naturally" in p^k individuals; it may occur as an autoantibody in PCH, in shich case it is a cold reactive IgG antibody and causes in vivo hemolysis.
NRBC	yes	?	?	yes	yes	cold			Anti-P + P_1P^k may occur in p individuals and can cause HTR and HDN.
NRBC	yes	some	rare	yes	occ	cold	rare	rare	M-N-cells may also be En(a−), in which case the cells are resistant to invasion by *P. falciparum* merozoites.
NRBC	yes	no	rare	yes	occ	cold	rare	rare	Anti-N-like antibodies may be produced in renal dialysis patients where the dialysis machine has been sterilized with formaldehyde.
RBC	some	yes	some	occ	yes	warm	yes	yes	
RBC	rare	yes	occ	occ	yes	warm	yes	yes	
RBC	no	yes	no	no	yes	warm	yes	yes	
NRBC	yes	some	some	yes	occ	cold	no	v.mild	Lu(a−b−) cells may result from inheritance of the recessive Lu gene or from the dominant In(Lu) gene. These cells are labile and hemolyze easily on storage. The antibody demonstrates a characteristic loose mixed-field agglutination pattern.
RBC	occ	yes	some	yes	yes	warm	yes	mild	

HEMATOLOGY/HEMOSTATIS REFERENCE RANGES

TESTS COMMONLY USED TO ASSESS ANEMIA

Test	Male	Female	Children
Serum iron	50–160 µg/dL	50–160 µg/dL	
Total iron binding capacity	250–1400 µg/dL	250–1400 µg/dL	
Percent iron saturation	20–55	20–55	
Ferritin	15–400 ng/mL	10–106 ng/dL	10–106 ng/dL
Serum vitamin B_{12}	200–850 pg/mL	200–850 pg/mL	
Serum folate	2.0–10.0 ng/mL	2.0–10.0 ng/mL	
RBC folate	>120 ng/mL	>120 ng/mL	
Hemoglobin A (electrophoresis)	95–100%	95–100%	
Hemoglobin A2 (electrophoresis)	0–3.5%	0–3.5%	
Hemoglobin F (electrophoresis)	0–2.0% (adult)	0–2.0% (adult)	Newborn 65–90% of total Hb 2 mo <46% 4 mo <10% 2 yr 2–5%
Haptoglobin	31–209 mg/dL	31–209 mg/dL	
Free hemoglobin, serum	0–10 mg/dL	0–10 mg/dL	

Reference Ranges

BODY FLUIDS

Cell count, cerebrospinal fluid	0–10 WBC/mm^3
Cell count, synovial fluid	WBC 0–200/mm^3 <25% neutrophils RBC 0 no crystals
Cell count, serious fluid	Dependent on body source; usually <1000 total WBC and/or 25% neutrophils

LYMPHOCYTE SUBSET/ADULTS

	%	Absolute
Lymphocytes, total	—	1400–3800 cells/mm^3
CD2	68–84	1200–2600 cells/mm^3
CD3	64–78	1000–2300 cells/mm^3
CD4	37–58	550–1600 cells/mm^3
CD8	14–32	200–700 cells/mm^3
H/S (CD4/CD8)	—	0.9–4.5
CD19	6–22	80–500 cells/mm^3
IgG	2–26	
IgM	4–18	
IgD	2–16	
IgA	0–5	
Kappa	7–25	
Lambda	4–18	

LYMPHOCYTE SUBSET/PEDIATRICS

	0–6 mo	6–12 mo	12–13 mo	18–24 mo	24–30 mo	30–36 mo	≥36 mo
Lymphocytes, total %	62–72	60–69	56–63	52–59	45–57	38–53	22–69
Lymphocytes, total absolute (cells/μL)	5395–7211	5284–6714	4943–5943	4431–5508	3855–5248	3315–5058	1622–5370
CD 4%	50–57	49–55	46–51	42–48	38–46	33–44	27–57
CD4 absolute (cells/μL)	2780–3908	2630–3499	2307–2864	1919–2472	1538–2213	1216–2009	562–2692
CD8%	8–31	8–31	8–31	8–31	8–31	8–31	14–34
CD8 absolute (cells/μL)	351–2479	351–2479	351–2479	351–2479	351–2479	351–2479	331–1445
CD2%	55–88	55–88	55–88	55–88	55–88	55–88	65–84
CD2 absolute (cells/μL)	3929–5275	3806–4881	3516–3868	3101–3868	2649–3639	2236–3463	1230–4074
CD3%	55–82	55–82	55–82	55–82	55–82	55–82	55–82
CD3 absolute (cells/μL)	3505–5009	3409–4575	3156–3899	2766–3508	2324–3295	1923–3141	1072–3890
CD19%	11–45	11–45	11–45	11–45	11–45	11–45	9–29
CD19 absolute	432–3345	432–3345	432–3345	432–3345	432–3345	432–3345	200–1259
Helper/Suppressor Ratio	1.2–6.2	1.2–6.2	1.2–6.2	1.2–6.2	1.2–6.2	1.2–6.2	0.98–3.24

HEMATOLOGY

Peripheral Blood

	Pediatric											Adult	
Test/Units	0–1d	2–4d	5–7d	8–14d	15–30d	1–2 mo	3–5 mo	6–11 mo	1–3 y	4–7 y	8–13 y	Male	Female
Hb g/dL	16.5–21.5	16.4–20.8	15.2–20.4	15.0–19.6	12.2–18.0	10.6–16.4	10.4–16.0	10.4–15.6	9.6–15.6	10.2–15.2	12.0–15.0	14.0–18.0	12.0–15.0
Hct %	48–68	18–68	50–64	46–62	38–53	32–50	35–51	35–51	34–48	34–48	35–49	40–54	35–49
WBC (X10^5/L)	9.0–37.0	8.0–24.0	5.0–21.0	5.0–21.0	5.0–21.0	6.0–18.0	6.0–18.0	6.0–18.0	5.5–17.5	5.0–17.0	4.5–13.5	4.5–11.5	4.5–11.5
RBC (X10^{12}/L)	4.10–6.10	4.36–5.96	4.20–5.80	4.00–5.60	3.20–5.00	3.40–5.00	3.65–5.05	3.60–5.20	3.40–5.20	4.00–5.20	4.00–5.40	4.60–6.00	4.00–5.40
MCV (IL)	95–125	98–118	100–120	95–115	93–113	83–107	83–107	78–102	76–92	78–94	80–94	80–94	80–94
MCH (pg)	30–42	30–42	30–42	30–42	28–40	27–37	25–35	23–31	23–31	23–31	26–32	26–32	26–32
MCHC (g/dL or %)	30–34	30–34	30–34	30–34	30–34	31–36	32–36	32–36	32–36	32–36	32–36	32–36	32–36
RDW (%)						11.5–14.5							
Bands %	4–14	3–11	3–9	1–8	0–5	0–5	0–5	0–5	0–5	0–5	0–5	0–5	0–5
Polys %	37–67	30–60	27–51	22–46	20–40	20–40	18–38	20–40	22–45	30–60	35–65	50–70	50–70
Lymphs %	18–38	16–46	24–54	30–62	41–61	42–72	45–75	48–78	37–73	29–65	23–53	18–42	18–42
Monos %	1–12	3–14	4–17	4–17	2–15	3–14	2–11	2–11	2–11	2–11	2–11	2–11	2–11
Eos %	1–4	1–5	2–5	1–5	1–5	1–4	1–4	1–4	1–4	1–4	1–4	1–3	1–3
Basos %	0–2	0–2	0–2	0–2	0–2	0–2	0–2	0–2	0–2	0–2	0–2	0–2	0–2
ANC (x10^8/L)	3.7–30.0	2.6–17.0	1.5–12.6	1.2–11.6	1.0–8.5	0.2–8.1	1.1–7.7	1.2–8.1	1.2–8.9	1.5–11.0	1.6–9.5	2.3–8.6	2.3–8.6
NRBC/ 100WBC	2–24	5–9	0–1	0	0	0	0	0	0	0	0	0	0
Retic %	1.8–5.8	1.3–4.7	0.2–1.4	0–1.0	0.2–1.0	0.8–2.8	0.5–1.5	0.5–1.5	0.5–1.5	0.5–1.5	0.5–1.5	0.5–1.5	0.5–1.5
Platelets (x10^9/L)						150–450							

Test	Reference Range	
Erythrocyte Sedimentation Rate (ESR) Westergren method	Male 0–50 years	1 hr = 0–15 mm
	Male 0–50 years	1 hr = 0–15 mm
	Female 0–50 years	1 hr = 0–15 mm
	Female 0–50 years	1 hr = 0–15 mm

Values from Indiana University Medical Center, Indianapolis, IN; current at time of print. Reference ranges may be method dependent, as well as affected by demographics, and must be determined and verified by each laboratory.

Abbreviations: Hb = hemoglobin; Hct = hematocrit; WBC = white blood cells; RBC = red blood cells; MCV = mean corpuscular volume; MCH = mean corpuscular hemoglobin; MCHC = mean corpuscular hemoglobin concentration; RDW = relative distribution width; Polys = polymorphonuclear neutrophils; Lymphs = lymphocytes; Monos = monocytes; Eos = eosinophils; Basos = basophils; ANC = absolute neutrophil count; NRBC = nucleated red blood cells; Retic = reticulocyte count.

Reprinted with permission from Rodak B: *Hematology: Clinical Principles and Applications, 2nd ed.* Philadelphia: Elsevier, 2002.

REFERENCE VALUES FOR *FREQUENTLY* ASSAYED CLINICAL CHEMISTRY ANALYTES

Analyte	Specimen	Reference Interval	
		Conventional Units	**Recommended SI Units**
Acid phosphatase (ACP) (ρ-Nitrophenylphosphate substrate)	S	Male 2.5–11.7 U/L Female 0.3–9.2 U/L	Male 1.2–19.5 × 10^{-8} katal/L Female 0.5–15.4 × 10^{-8} katal/L
Alanine aminotransferase (ALT)	S	6–37 UL	1–6.2 × 10^{-7} katal/L
Albumin	S	3.5–5.5 g/dL	35–55 g/L
Alkaline phosphatase (ALP)	S	30–90 U/L (30°C)	30–95 U/L Bowers and McComb
Ammonia	P	19–60 µg/dL	11–35 mmol/L
Amylase	S U	60–180 SU/dL 35–400 U/hr	95–290 U/L
Anion gap	Calculated		10–20 mmol/L
Aspartate aminotransferase (AST)	S	5–30 U/L	8.3–50 × 10^{-8} katal/L
Bicarbonate (HCO_3)	WB	22–26 mmol/L	
Bilirubin	S	Total 0.2–1.0 mg/dL Conjugated 0–0.2 mg/dL	3–17 µmol/L 0–3 µmol/L
Blood Gases (arterial) pH Pco_2 Po_2	WB	 7.35–7.45 35–45 mmHg 80–110 mmol/L	
Blood urea nitrogen (BUN)	S	7–18 mg/dL	2.5–6.4 mmol/L urea
Calcium (Ca^+), (total)	S	Adult 8.6–10.0 mg/dL Child 8.6–10.6 mg/dL	2.15–2.50 mmol/L 2.15–2.65 mmol/L
Calcium (Ionized)	S	Adult 1.6–5.3 mg/dL Neonate 4.8–5.9 mg/dL	1.16–1.32 mmol/L 1.20–1.48 mmol/L
Carbon dioxide (CO_2), (total)	P, S	22–29 mEq/L	22–29 mmol/L
Chloride (Cl^-)	S U (24 hr)	98–106 mEq/L 110–250 mEq/L	98–107 mmol/L 110–250 mmol/L
Cholesterol (total)	S	140–200 mg/dL	3.6–5.2 mmol/L
Cortisol	P	Morning 5–23 µg/dL Evening 3–16 µg/dL	221–552 mmol/L <138 mmol/L
Creatine kinase (CK)	S	Male 15–160 U/L Female 15–130 U/L	0.25–2.67 × 10^{-6} katal/L 0.25–2.17 × 10^{-6} katal/L
Creatine kinase isoenzyme-MB (CK-MB)	S	<6% of total CK	
Creatinine	S	Male 0.6–1.2 mg/dL Female 0.5–1.1 mg/dL	53–106 mmol/L 44–97 mmol/L
Creatinine clearance	U	Male 97–137 mL/min/173 m^2 Female 88–128 mL/min/1.73 m^2	53–106 mmol/L 44–97 mmol/L
Gamma-glutamyl transferase (GGT)	S	Male 6–45 U/L Female 5–30 U/L	10–75 × 10^{-6} katal/L 8–50 × 10^{-6} katal/L

Analyte	Specimen	Reference Interval	
		Conventional Units	Recommended SI Units
Gamma immunoglobulins	S	IgG 800–1200 mg/dL IgA 70–312 mg/dL IgM 50–280 mg/dL IgD 0.5–2.8 mg/dL IgE 0.01–0.06 mg/dL	IgG 8–12 g/L IgA 0.7–3.12 g/L IgM 0.5–2.8 g/L IgD 0.005–0.200 g/L IgE 0.1–0.6 g/L
Glucose (fasting)	P CSF	Fasting 70–110 mg/dL 10–70 mg/dL	3.9–6.0 mmol/L 2.2–3.9 mmol/L
Glycosylated hemoglobin (GHb)	P	4.5–8.0	
High-density lipoprotein (HDL) cholesterol	S	Male 29–60 mg/dL Female 38–75 mg/dL	0.75–1.60 mmol/L 1.00–1.94 mmol/L
Iron	S	Male 65–170 µg/dL Female 50–170 µg/dL	
Lactate dehydrogenase (LD)	S	(L → P) 100–225 U/L (P → L) 80–280 U/L	

Lactate dehydrogenase
  isoenzymes
  (as percentage of total)
	S	LD-1 14–26%
		LD-2 29–39%
		LD-3 20–26%
		LD-4 8–16%
		LD-5 6–16%	

Lipase	S	0.0–1.0 U/mL	
Magnesium (Mg^{2+})	S U	1.2–2.1 mEq/L 6.0–10.0 mEq/24 hr	0.63–1.00 mmol/L 3.00–5.00 mmol/24 hr
Osmolality Urine-serum ratio	S U (24 hr)	275–295 mOsmol/kg 300–900 mOsmol/kg 1.0–3.0	
Phosphate	S	2.7–4.5 mg/dL	0.87–1.45 mmol/L
Potassium (K^+)	S U (24 hr)	3.4–5.0 mEq/L Neonate 3.7–5.9 mEq/L 25–125 mEq/d	3.4–5.0 mmol/L 3.7–5.9 mmol/L 25–125 mmol/d
Protein (total)	S CSF	6.5–8.3 g/dL 0.5% of plasma	65–83 g/L
Sodium (Na^+)	S U (24 h) CSF	135–145 mEq/L 40–220 mEq/L 138–150 mEq/L	135–145 mmol/L 40–220 mmol/L 138–150 mmol/L
Thyroid-stimulating hormone (TSH)	S	0.5–5.0 µU/mL	
Thyroxine (T_4)	S	4.5–13.0 µg/dL	58–167 mmol/L
Triglycerides	S	67–157 mg/dL	0.11–2.15 mmol/L
Uric acid	S	Male 3.5–7.2 mg/dL Female 2.6–6.0 mg/dL	208–428 µmol/L 155–357 µmol/L

Values may vary according to method and population; values for enzymes are at 37°C unless otherwise noted.

Abbreviations: S = serum; P = plasma; U = urine; CSF = cerebrospinal fluid; WB = whole blood.

Reprinted with permission from Bishop M, Engelkirk J, Fody E: *Clinical Chemistry, Principles, Procedures, Correlations, 4th ed.* Philadelphia: Lippincott, 2000.

Test	Abbreviation	Specimen Considerations	Clinical Correlation
Drug Monitoring			
Amikacin		Do not use gel barrier tube; centrifuge and separate within 1 hour	Broad-spectrum antibiotic
Carbamazepine (Tegretol)		Do not use gel barrier tube	Mood-stabilizing in bipolar affective discorder
Digoxin (Lanoxin)		Do not use gel barrier tube	Heart stimulant
Dilantin (Phenytoin)		Do not use gel barrier tube	Treatment of epilepsy
Gentamcin		Do not use gel barrier tube	Broad-spectrum antibiotic
Lithium		Do not use gel barrier tube; should be drawn 8–12 hours after dose administered	Manic depression medication
Phenobarbitol (barbiturates)		Do not use gel barrier tube	Anticonvulsant for seizures
Salicylates (aspirin)		Do not use gel barrier tube	Evaluation of therapy
Theophylline		Do not use gel barrier tube	Asthma medication
Tobramycin		Do not use gel barrier tube	Broad-spectrum antibiotic
Vancomycin		Do not use gel barrier tube	Broad-spectrum antibiotic
Ferritin		Refrigerate serum	Hemochromatosis, iron deficiency
Gamma-glutamyl transpeptidase	GGTP		Liver function
Gastrin		Overnight fasting is required; separate serum from cells within 1 hour after collection; freeze serum	Stomach disorders
Glucose	FBS - fasting blood sugar; RBS - random blood sugar	Separate from cells within 1 hour or use gray-top tube	Diabetes, hypoglycemia
Glycosylated hemoglobin	Hgb A_k	Lavender tube	Monitoring diabetes mellitus
Glucose-6-phosphate dehydrogenase	G-6-PD	Lavender tube; do not freeze	Drug-induced anemias
Hemoglobin electrophoresis		Refrigerate; whole blood; do not spin	Hemoglobinopathies and thalassemia
HLA typing A and B		Yellow-top (ACD) tubes; do not freeze or refrigerate; ethnic origin must be included	Disease association, bone marrow, platelet capability, liver or heart transplant
Human chorionic gonadotropin	HCG		Pregnancy, testicular cancer
Immunoglobulins IgA, IgG, IgM			Measurement of proteins capable of becoming antibodies, chronic liver disease. myeloma

Test	Abbreviation	Specimen Considerations	Clinical Correlation
Iron, total	Fe	Drawn in AM, should be fasting; avoid hemolysis	Iron toxicity or deficiency
Lactate/lactic acid		Plasma-gray top; do not use a tourniquet during phlebotomy or allow patient to clench their fist	Glucose metabolism
Lactic dehydrogenase	LDH	Serum, avoid hemolysis—do not freeze	Cardiac injury and other muscle damage
Lead	Pb	Royal blue EDTA or tan-top lead-free tube; do not centrifuge	Lead toxicity
Lipase		Refrigerate serum	Pancreatic disease
Lipoproteins— high-density	HDL	Must be fasting a minimum of 12 hours	Evaluates lipid disorders and coronary artery disease risk
low-density	LDL	Must be fasting a minimum of 12 hours	Evaluates lipid disorders and coronary artery disease risk
Magnesium	Mg		Mineral metabolism, kidney function
Phosphorus	P		Thyroid function, bone disorders, kidney disease
Prostate-specific antigen	PSA	Refrigerate serum; draw before rectal examination or biopsy	Prostate cancer
Serum protein electrophoresis	SPEP or PEP		Abnormal protein detection
Sweat electrolytes (iontophoresis)	Sweat chloride	Fluid collected is sweat	Cystic fibrosis
Thyroid studies	T_3, T_4, TSH		Hyper- or hypothyroid conditions
Total iron binding capacity and Fe	TIBC and Fe	Drawn in AM, should be fasting	
Triglycerides		Fasting 12–14 hours is required	Atherosclerosis and heart disease
Troponin			Marker for myocardial infarc
Uric acid			Gout
Zinc	Zn	Royal blue, no additive	Liver dysfunction

Types of collection tubes: Red, nonadditive (do not mix); SST, inert gel and silica; Green, sodium heparin, lithium heparin, ammonia heparin; Gray, sodium fluoride, potassium oxalate; Royal blue, free of trace element, can be red label, green label, lavender label.

Reprinted with permission as adapted from McCall RL, Tankersley CM: *Phlebotomy Essentials, 2nd ed.* Philadelphia: Lippincott, 1998, in Bishop M; Engelkirk J, Fody E: *Clinical Chemistry: Principles, Procedures, Correlations, 4th ed.* Philadelphia: Lippincott, 2000.

▶ APPENDIX B

PATIENT: ROBERTA BANKS

Study Questions A

1. *Clinical Symptoms:* Tired, weak

    Background History: Non-Hodgkin's lymphoma, receiving chemotherapy

2. Hemoglobin and hematocrit

4. a. Both hemoglobin and hematocrit are below the reference ranges.

    b. The patient has anemia.

Study Questions B

2. a. Group O Rh (D) negative. Yes, there are no discrepancies detected.

Patient Cells with			Patient Serum with	
Anti-A	Anti-B	Anti-D	A_1 cells	B cells
0	0	0	+	4+

    b. 3-cell antibody screen shows antibodies present.

	IS	37°C	AHG
Screening Cell I:	0	0	3+
Screening Cell II:	0	0	3+
Screening Cell III:	0	0	3+

    2-unit red blood cell compatibility test: 2 of 2 units incompatible.

    c. An antibody panel and a direct antiglobulin test (DAT) should be performed next.

    All panel cells, along with the auto control, react 3+ at the AHG phase of testing.

A second panel shows 3+ AHG reactivity with all panel cells except one.

Since the patient has not been recently transfused, a warm autoadsorption can be performed on the patient's serum. This autoadsorbed serum can then be tested against the same panel cells for comparison.

An eluate can be performed on the red blood cells of the patient. The eluate can then be tested against the same panel cells for comparison.

In this patient, antibody panel test results with autoadsorbed serum are as follows: Certain panel cells are nonreactive with the autoadsorbed serum. The reactive panel cells show 3+ reactivity at the AHG phase of testing.

The antibody panel test results with eluate are as follows: All panel cells show 3+ reactivity at the AHG phase of testing.

d. The patient has warm autoantibodies that show an anti-e specificity. The patient also has an underlying allo-anti-K. The eluate studies reveal the presence of a panagglutinin.

3. The auto-anti-e and the allo-anti-K have been confirmed and all other clinically significant antibodies have been ruled out. The case can be completed by phenotyping the patient for the presence or absence of the e and K antigens.

Patient phenotyping results:

e antigen: Positive

K antigen: Negative

4. Because of the presence of warm autoantibodies, it is best not to transfuse the patient unless it is absolutely needed to increase oxygen-carrying capacity. If the patient must be transfused, the products must be ABO/Rh group O negative and K antigen negative. Even though the autoantibody shows an anti-e specificity, the transfusion of e-antigen-negative red blood cells is probably not necessary. The compatibility test result for these products will be incompatible. In these transfusion cases, it is best to transfuse the products that are the least incompatible (most compatible) with the serum of the patient.

CASE SUMMARY

PATIENT: ROBERTA BANKS

The patient developed warm autoimmune hemolytic anemia along with her non-Hodgkin's lymphoma. The patient's serum revealed an autoantibody (anti-e) and an alloantibody (anti-K). The eluate prepared from the patient's red blood cells revealed a panagglutinin, which is an antibody that is capable of agglutinating all red blood cells.

The hemoglobin/hematocrit of the patient is declining. The best situation would be for the patient not to require a transfusion. In this case, the anemia was controlled with corticosteroids and the patient did not require a transfusion.

If the patient did require a transfusion, the best product to provide would be an ABO/Rh group O negative red blood cell product that is K-antigen negative. A red blood cell product that is also e-antigen negative will probably not survive any better when transfused to the patient, even though this product may be compatible with the patient in the laboratory. Eliminating the need for the patient to receive e-antigen-negative red blood cells makes the process faster and easier in providing the patient with products. In this case, the blood bank would probably have to contact the rare donor registry in order to obtain red blood cell products that are D-antigen negative, e-antigen negative, and K-antigen negative.

ANSWERS TO LEARNING ACTIVITIES

PATIENT: JOAN F. CANALY

Study Questions A

1. *Clinical Symptoms*: Hyperpigmentation, decreased blood pressure, weight loss, severe fatigue

    Background History: Hypothyroidism

2. CBC, UA, *thyroid profile, *ACTH, *aldosterone, *cortisol, CMP

    * = Tests that correlate with presenting symptoms

4. Increased potassium and TSH and markedly increased ACTH concentrations

    Decreased calcium, aldosterone, and cortisol concentrations

5. a. Increased potassium and markedly increased ACTH concentrations

    Decreased aldosterone and cortisol concentrations

    b. ACTH: 4492 pg/mL (9–52 pg/mL)

    c. Primary adrenal insufficiency; Addison's disease

    d. Yes; all of Ms. Canaly's presenting symptoms are consistent with a diagnosis of Addison's disease.

6. The following result suggests that her hypothyroidism is not controlled:

    TSH: 5.25 (0.49–4.67μU/mL)

Study Questions B

1. In normal individuals, ACTH is released from the pituitary gland as a result of stimulus from CRH released from the hypothalamus gland. The ACTH then regulates the adrenal cortex to release cortisol. Increased levels of cortisol then act on the hypothalamus and pituitary glands to reduce ACTH production, which lowers cortisol concentrations. When cortisol concentrations drop below a certain level, the hypothalamus releases CRH, which stimulates the pituitary to release ACTH, which stimulates the adrenal cortex to release cortisol.

2. Aldosterone is a mineralocorticoid produced by the adrenal cortex that controls the balance between sodium, potassium, and chloride concentrations. A decreased aldosterone concentration will decrease sodium and chloride concentrations while increasing potassium concentrations.

3. Diurnal variation is especially pronounced in ACTH and cortisol secretion patterns. The peak concentrations of ACTH and cortisol are seen at 8 A.M. and the lowest concentrations at 4 P.M. The reference ranges of these analytes are significantly different at 8 A.M. and 4 P.M., so it is critical that the time of specimen collection be known in order to make an appropriate interpretation of test results.

4. a. Primary adrenal insufficiency

    b. Increased concentrations of ACTH indicate that the pituitary gland is trying to stimulate release of cortisol from the adrenal cortex, but the adrenal gland is not able to respond.

    c. There is a family history of congestive heart failure. Persons taking steroid replacements are at increased cardiovascular risk. It is important to get a baseline result on this patient in order to monitor her response to long-term steroid therapy.

5. Decreased blood pressure

6. In an Addisonian crisis, the patient is exposed to a dramatically decreased concentration of cortisol, which results in a serious emergency condition. Sodium and glucose concentrations drop, and potassium concentrations rise. An Addisonian crisis is usually a result of stress, surgery, severe infection, or acute fluid loss. Death can result from circulatory collapse unless prompt treatment is initiated.

7. Schmidt's syndrome is a combination of abnormalities that includes hypothyroidism and Addison's disease, usually of autoimmune origin. The average age of onset is 30, and it may occur in combination with hyperglycemia. It is considered a polyendocrine deficiency disorder.

CASE SUMMARY

PATIENT: JOAN CANALY

Ms. Canaly was seen in her primary-care physician's office with initial symptoms of hyperpigmentation, fatigue, weight loss, and light-headedness. She had been previously diagnosed with primary hypothyroidism and was being treated with Synthroid. A significant finding on physical examination was hypotension. The pigmentation suggested an increased secretion of ACTH, which was confirmed by the laboratory with an extremely increased concentration of 4492 pg/mL (the reference range being 9–52 pg/mL). MRI scans of the pituitary gland and a CT scan of the adrenal glands revealed no abnormalities in either.

The patient was referred to an endocrinologist, who confirmed the diagnosis of Schmidt's syndrome, a disease characterized by hypothyroidism and primary adrenal insufficiency with an average age of onset of 30. The patient was treated with mineralocorticoid replacements and dexamethasone to reduce skin pigmentations. Close follow-up by both an endocrinologist and the primary-care physician is necessary to ensure proper treatment in controlling the hormonal abnormalities. After one episode of edema and shortness of breath due to excessive medication, the patient currently appears to be successfully controlling her condition.

Addison's disease can be adequately controlled with appropriate medications and diligent monitoring of each patient's condition. It is important that the patient and all health-care providers be aware of this condition. Since cortisol secretion significantly increases in times of illness, stress, infection, injury, or surgery, routine doses of steroids should be increased during these times.

ANSWERS TO LEARNING ACTIVITIES

PATIENT: MICHAEL CARPENTER

Study Questions A

1. *Clinical Symptoms:* Fatigue, jaundice

   Background History: Type 2 diabetes mellitus, hyperlipidemia

2. Liver profile: TP, Alb, Glob, A/G, ALP, *T. bili, *D. bili, AST, *ALT; lipid profile: Chol, *HDL, LDL, Trig, *LDL/HDL ratio; GGT; ferritin; *HgbA1c; CBC

   * = Tests that correlate with presenting symptoms

4. No

5. T. bili, D. bili, ALT

6.   Yes. Jaundice is due to the increase in bilirubin concentrations, especially the increased direct bilirubin. Direct bilirubin is water soluble and as such deposits easily in the tissues. It is especially noticeable in the sclera of the eyes and the mucous membranes.

Study Questions B

1.   a. T. bili, D. bili, ALT

     b. The lack of immunologic markers for hepatitis A, B, or C indicates that Mr. Carpenter does not have infectious hepatitis caused by these viruses.

     c. Any liver disease that increases hepatic enzymes and bilirubin concentrations will give negative results on a hepatitis panel. One should consider diseases such as toxic hepatitis, other hepatitis viruses (D to H), Wilson's disease, hemochromatosis, $alpha_1$-antitrypsin deficiencies, hepatic tumors, fulminant hepatic failure, and primary biliary cirrhosis.

     d. Increases in ferritin concentration due to release of the stored ferritin from damaged hepatocytes occur in hepatic injury and can be used as an indicator of the degree of hepatic damage. While this patient's symptoms are consistent with hemochromatosis, a condition that also increases ferritin concentrations, the normal results on this patient's CBC rules out hemochromatosis.

2.   a. Glucose and hemoglobin A1c concentrations

     b. Hemoglobin A1c concentrations reflect the mean glucose concentration that red blood cells have been exposed to in vivo for the past 8 to 10 weeks. It is an indicator of long-term glycemic control, whereas glucose concentrations reflect only the glucose concentration of the past few hours.

3.   Glipizide, 5 mg twice per day. This oral medication acts to stimulate the release of insulin from the beta cells in the pancreas.

4.   No. The HgbA1c concentration remains consistently elevated despite the oral medication. If the patient is not diligent in his dietary restrictions, the action of the medication may not be sufficient to control glucose concentrations.

5.   Continue to monitor serum glucose and HgbA1c concentrations and continue to encourage the patient to adhere to his prescribed diet and exercise program.

6.   The chronic hyperglycemia of diabetes is associated with long-term damage to various organs, especially the eyes, kidneys, nerves, heart, and blood vessels.

7. a. The action of Lipitor should decrease triglyceride concentrations by up to 40 percent. Control of Mr. Carpenter's diabetes also will decrease triglyceride concentrations.

    b. Yes. It primarily increases the risk of the development of vascular diseases and the development and progression of coronary heart disease. Deposits of lipid can occur in any organ, but they are most critical when they accumulate in the vessels of the heart, liver, and kidney, resulting in restriction of blood flow, initiation of clot formation, or circulatory obstructions. Plaque composed of lipid can result in CVAs and infarctions of many organs and systems.

8. Epidemiologic studies have identified a number of risk factors for coronary artery disease, including elevation of serum lipids. Development of atherosclerotic disease is a complicated process involving various lipid-containing particles. It has long been recognized that cardiac risk factors tend to cluster in individual patients. A combination of insulin resistance, high triglyceride levels, and the presence of small, dense, atherogenic low-density lipoprotein cholesterol particles is highly predictive of atherosclerosis. It is also recognized that low levels of high-density lipoprotein (HDL) cholesterol particles are associated with increased cardiovascular risk, especially in women and diabetic patients.

9. Among the studies that have looked at HDL cholesterol levels and CAD, the Framingham Heart Study showed low HDL levels to be an independent risk factor for CAD. Specifically, there was a 10 percent increase in CAD for each 4-mg/dL decrease in HDL. In addition, angiographic studies have shown a correlation between low HDL cholesterol levels and an increased number of diseased coronary arteries

10. a. Yes, Mr. Carpenter has all of the hallmarks of the metabolic syndrome.

    b. Significantly elevated risk of CAD, which would be likely to result in myocardial infarction and/or stroke.

    c. Yes; increased serum lipids increase the likelihood of lipid being deposited in the liver.

11. No critical laboratory evaluations were omitted.

12. For the most part, the use of the laboratory in this case was appropriate. Multiple determinations of liver function studies, lipid profiles, and HgbA1c are all appropriate to follow Mr. Carpenter's response to treatment for his diabetes and increased lipids. In retrospect, the iron study and ferritin concentration were not essential to Mr. Carpenter's diagnosis, although the ferritin concentration could have given information regarding the degree of hepatocyte damage, if that process had been occurring. Since there is no hepatic destruction in Mr. Carpenter, there is no need for this laboratory assessment.

CASE SUMMARY

PATIENT: MICHAEL CARPENTER

Mr. Carpenter is a 35-year-old white male with three distinct, but related, medical conditions. He has developed Type 2 diabetes mellitus that is not being adequately controlled by diet, exercise, and oral hypoglycemic agents. His serum glucose concentration has remained between 170 and 290 mg/dL over the period for which we have his medical record. Hemoglobin A1c concentrations reflect this hyperglycemic state. The patient was advised of his need to be diligent in adhering to his low-carbohydrate diet and regular exercise and was placed on an increased dose of Glipizide.

The second condition identified in Mr. Carpenter is hyperlipidemia. The lipid profile at the first office visit showed extremely elevated triglycerides, moderate increases in total and LDL cholesterol, and decreased concentrations of HDL cholesterol. Lipitor normalized the triglycerides and cholesterol concentrations, lowering his risk for CAD.

The patient initiated this office visit as a result of increasing fatigue and slight jaundice. Referral to a gastroenterologist for abdominal ultrasound found diffuse fatty infiltration of the liver.

These three conditions are certainly related, as the carbohydrate intolerance results in release of lipid for an energy source, and the familial elevations of lipid further complicate the situation. Excess fatty material is then collected in the liver and replaces normally functioning liver tissue with fat deposits. This results in lowered liver capacity and function, as is seen in Mr. Carpenter's hepatic profiles.

This patient requires aggressive therapeutic intervention to control his diabetes and hyperlipidemia in order to prevent further deterioration of liver functions.

Mr. Carpenter is a young man to have these conditions and should be counseled on the benefits of strict control of his diet for carbohydrate and fat consumption, exercise, weight reduction, and appropriate drug therapy to prevent irreversible heart and liver damage in the future. If his current path is not altered, severe health problems loom ahead.

ANSWERS TO LEARNING ACTIVITIES

PATIENT: DEIDRA CARTER

Study Questions A

1. *Clinical Symptoms:* Pain in left upper leg.

   Background History: Automobile accident victim. Suffered injury. No other significant or related medical history. No history of transfusion or pregnancy; no medications. Two 500-mg aspirin tablets to treat a headache 3 h prior.

2.   *Hemoglobin and *hematocrit

   * = Tests that correlate with presenting symptoms

4.   a. Low hemoglobin and low hematocrit

   b. The patient is either anemic or bleeding.

Study Questions B

2.   The patient is Rh(D) positive; however, an ABO discrepancy is detected.

3.   The patient has a forward ABO type of A and a reverse ABO type of O; therefore, an ABO discrepancy exists. To resolve this discrepancy, test the cells of the patient with anti-A_1 lectin (*Dolichos biflorus*) and the serum of the patient with A_2 cells.

4.   The patient is a subgroup of the A blood type. The patient has the blood type A_2 with anti-A_1 present in the serum.

5.   The A_2 blood type of the patient has been confirmed. In order to confirm the presence of the anti-A_1 antibody in the patient, additional antigen-positive and antigen-negative cells are tested with the serum of the patient. The negative three-cell antibody screen rules out other potential patient alloantibodies. Testing the patient's serum with two additional cells of the A_1 phenotype (if the test results are positive) and two additional cells of the A_2 phenotype (if the test results are negative) would statistically confirm the presence of the anti-A_1 in the patient's serum.

6.   To determine what RBC products to provide the patient, the clinical significance of the anti-A_1 must be assessed. This can be done by applying the prewarm technique on the reverse type of the patient.

7.   Group O red blood cells or group A_2 red blood cells that have been phenotyped and found to be negative for the A_1 antigen. Because anti-A_1 demonstrated reactivity at 37°C, the antibody can be considered clinically significant.

8.   a. 40   c. 8

   b. 8   d. 0

CASE SUMMARY

PATIENT: DEIDRA CARTER

This patient presented with an ABO discrepancy. The 2+ result in the test between the patient serum and reagent A_1 cells gave a good indication as to which test result was unexpected. In this case, the patient had an unexpected positive result in her serum tests.

Since the antibody screen on the patient was negative, the presence of an unexpected ABO antibody was investigated. The suspected antibody identification was anti-A_1. Only non-A_1 individuals can produce this antibody. In order to place the patient in a non-A_1 subgroup, a test of the patient's cells with anti-A_1 lectin (*Dolichos biflorus*) was performed. Only those cells that react with properly diluted *Dolichos biflorus* can be placed in the A_1 blood type. The failure of the patient's cells to react with this reagent shows that the patient belongs to a non-A_1 subgroup. The most probable subgroup is A_2. The confirmation of the suspected anti-A_1 was achieved by testing the patient's serum with three examples from each of the following red blood cell phenotypes: A_1, A_2, and O. If the serum reacts with only the three A_1 cells and not the A_2 or O cells, then the antibody can be identified as anti-A_1.

Once the antibody has been identified as anti-A_1, the clinical significance of the antibody must then be determined. Anti-A_1 usually reacts at temperatures below 30°C and is considered clinically insignificant. This would allow the patient to receive a transfusion of A_1 red cells without having much of a transfusion reaction risk. If the anti-A_1 demonstrates reactivity at 37°C, then the antibody can be considered clinically significant. The patient should receive a transfusion of only A_2 or O red cells.

The clinical significance of the antibody is demonstrated by performing the prewarm technique. This technique warms the patient's antibody and the reagent red cells to 37°C prior to their incubation together. A negative prewarm technique shows that the antibody does not react at 37°C and is clinically insignificant. A positive prewarm technique shows that the antibody does react at 37°C and should be considered clinically significant.

ANSWERS TO LEARNING ACTIVITIES

PATIENT: ROBERT CHOWNING

Study Questions A

A.   1. *Clinical Symptoms:* Productive cough, joint pain, diarrhea

   Background History: Sore throat 2 weeks prior, fever, nausea and vomiting for 2 days

2.   a. *Complete blood count (CBC), glucose, *BUN, *electrolytes, *sputum culture and susceptibility studies

   * = Tests that correlate with presenting symptoms

   b. As a screening test, CBC is an indicator of many disease conditions; it provides the physician with an overview of the patient's ability to fight disease and allows monitoring of the body's ability to respond to therapy. An elevated WBC, for example, is a marker for infection.

Serum electrolytes determine the patient's state of hydration. Because the patient has experienced vomiting and diarrhea for several days, he may be suffering from dehydration. BUN is a kidney function test.

4. a. Mr. Chowning's WBC count is elevated and the peripheral blood smear differential shows neutrophilia. His platelet count is also markedly decreased. Increased WBCs with predominantly polymorphonuclear cells (PMNs) usually suggests the presence of an infectious process. Abnormal platelet counts may accompany a wide variety of diseases and conditions. A patient with a platelet count of less than 150,000/μL is generally considered thrombocytopenic, although bleeding episodes may not occur unless the platelet count falls below 50,000/μL.

    b. The chemistry results, overall, are unremarkable, with the exception of the electrolytes. Na^{2+} and K^+ are below the acceptable range, an imbalance that may have resulted from loss of fluids due to diarrhea and vomiting.

    Blood urea nitrogen (BUN), although outside the normal parameters, is only slightly elevated. The anion gap is also increased. Both tests are indicators of renal function.

    c. Fever is part of the body's immune response and manifests as a result of the release of interleukin-1 (IL-1), interleukin-2 (IL-2), and tumor necrosis factor (TNF) from white blood cells, especially macrophages. Acute-phase proteins are also secreted as a response to an assault on the host. An elevated WBC is an indicator of an infectious process, especially when accompanied by neutrophilia. The electrolyte results indicate the patient's state of hydration, while the BUN and creatinine test the kidney function. In this patient, the results indicate a state of dehydration. Fever can be induced by most infectious processes, either systemic or local, or may be due to neoplasms and other vascular-collagen diseases.

    The patient presented with cough and fever, possibly manifestations of a lower respiratory tract infection. The increased WBC with neutrophilia and fever is consistent with this infectious process. The patient's admitting diagnosis was pneumonia. Electrolytes and renal function test results correlated with the patient's history of vomiting and diarrhea for several days.

5. a. A sputum culture was requested and a direct smear performed. Culture of the sputum may reveal the etiology of the patient's cough. The clinician suspected pneumonia, a lower respiratory tract infection. The sputum direct smear was performed to determine if a proper specimen was submitted. Because sputum samples contain normal respiratory flora, it is important to assess the acceptability of the sample. If the direct smear shows inflammatory cells and few epithelial

cells, this indicates the presence of an infectious process and also indicates that the sample came from the lower respiratory tract. If epithelial cells are predominant, this is indicative of oral mucosal contamination and is not a representative sample, and so culture interpretation may be misleading. The predominant organism in the sample should also be observed on the direct smear and reported.

b. The sputum direct smear shows numerous white blood cells, primarily PMNs, rare squamous epithelial cells, and a predominance of gram-positive cocci in pairs and short chains. The direct smear results indicate that the sputum sample was representative of the lower respiratory tract secretions and is acceptable for culture. These are significant findings, and the clinician should be alerted. The presence of a large amount of PMNs indicates that an infectious process is occurring in the particular body site where the sample was taken. In Mr. Chowning's case, the predominance of a single morphotype suggests the presence of infection by that organism rather than colonization.

c. Normal respiratory flora were recovered from the sputum culture, although the direct smear showed the predominance of a single morphotype that resembles *Streptococcus pneumoniae*. These findings suggest that the respiratory syndrome may be of viral origin or the result of a partially treated bacterial infection. Because the patient has been on antibiotic therapy prior to specimen collection, the etiologic agent may have been inhibited from producing growth in culture. It is therefore important to perform sputum direct smears and evaluate the significance of the microscopic results. In this case, the culture results do not correlate and are not consistent with the direct smear findings. The clinician must be alerted to these findings so that further investigation is performed.

Study Questions B

1. a. Blood cultures three times 1 h apart; stool culture and examination for ova and parasites; repeat CBC, BUN, electrolytes, creatinine; PT; APTT; fibrinogen; platelet count; lumbar puncture for cerebrospinal fluid (CSF) studies: CSF cell count and differential, CSF glucose and protein, CSF direct smear and culture

b. Within hours of his admission to the hospital, the patient developed petechial lesions that eventually became necrotic. This clinical presentation may appear during the initial stages of disseminated intravascular coagulation (DIC), when platelets and coagulation proteins are consumed. In DIC, the fibrinolytic system is activated. Microvascular thrombosis occurs, then hemorrhage and necrosis develop, eventually resulting in peripheral gangrene.

Stool culture, examination for ova and parasites, and test for occult blood were performed to detect the presence of enteric pathogens that may be causing the watery diarrhea. Because the patient remained febrile, blood cultures were requested to determine the presence of bacteremia or other forms of systemic infection.

c. Headache, fever, stiff neck, and vomiting are classic symptoms of meningeal infection. The patient also remained febrile.

3. a. The results of the coagulation studies show indications of DIC. Although DIC may occur in various clinical conditions, it is often associated with septicemia, particularly in gram-negative sepsis. However, any microorganism can initiate DIC, including gram-positive organisms. Cell-specific membrane components of microorganisms, such as endotoxin or lipopolysaccharide of gram-negative bacteria, may activate the coagulation syndrome. Other initiators that may induce DIC include superantigen exotoxins of gram-positive organisms, all of which activate cytokine complex.

b. The chemistry and hematology laboratory findings supported the clinical diagnosis of meningococcal meningitis. The CSF cell count was abnormal, protein was elevated, and glucose was decreased. Coagulopathy developed as a result of sepsis.

4. a. The CSF Gram-stained direct smear showed numerous white blood cells and intracellular gram-negative diplococci. When present in body fluids, white blood cells indicate the presence of infection. Finding gram-negative intracellular diplococci in the CSF is significant, and even life-threatening.

b. The culture grew gram-negative diplococci, later identified as *Neisseria meningitidis*, one of the most common causes of bacterial meningitis, a life-threatening infection. The isolate was consistent with the direct smear findings.

c. The most serious complication of meningococcemia is DIC, which can be life-threatening. This potentially fatal disease may follow a progressive course that includes hemorrhages in the adrenal glands, referred to as Waterhouse-Friderichsen syndrome, and subcutaneous hemorrhages that result from DIC. Individuals who show complement deficiency (C5 to C9) are at risk for recurrent meningococcal disease and associated complications.

d. This patient suffered from DIC as a complication of meningococcemia. Treatment of DIC requires an aggressive but appropriate regimen to stop the triggering mechanism or the causative disease process.

CASE SUMMARY

PATIENT: ROBERT CHOWNING

Mr. Chowning, a 30-year-old Hispanic male, presented with initial symptoms of a respiratory type of infection, reporting soreness of throat and cough, followed by fever. He also complained of nausea and vomiting with watery diarrhea. He experienced generalized malaise, weakness, and myalgia. Because of the primary clinical presentation, the patient was presumptively diagnosed with pneumonia. The clinician requested a sputum culture. The sputum culture yielded primarily normal respiratory flora, although the sputum direct smear indicated purulence and predominance of morphotypes resembling *Streptococcus pneumoniae*, an opportunistic respiratory pathogen. His respiratory syndrome might have a viral origin or be attributable to a partially treated infection because he received antibiotic therapy with amoxicillin prior to his admission to the hospital.

Stool culture, examination for ova and parasites, and test for occult blood were performed to detect the presence of enteric pathogens that might be causing the watery diarrhea. These laboratory tests also produced negative findings.

The CBC results on admission showed an increased white blood cell count (WBC) with elevated PMNs. These findings indicate the presence of an infectious process, which could be of bacterial etiology. Chemistry test results were insignificant, except for the electrolytes, which showed an imbalance, an indication of mild dehydration as a result of vomiting and diarrheal episodes.

The day following his admission to the facility, Mr. Chowning developed a rash all over his body that later progressed into necrotic lesions, especially on his face, chest, and extremities, such as fingers and toes. Mr. Chowning's illness worsened, with sustained fever, and showed neurologic symptoms that included hallucination and lethargy. Lumbar puncture was performed, and the CSF studies showed evidence of an acute bacterial meningitis. Coagulation studies indicated an ensuing disseminated intravascular coagulation (DIC). Tests performed on the CSF revealed the presence of gram-negative intracellular diplococci, resembling *Neisseria* species. The isolate was later identified as *Neisseria meningitidis*. This finding was consistent with the blood culture isolates. CSF glucose concentration was decreased, and CSF protein concentration was elevated. WBC count and differential on the CSF also showed increased leukocytosis and neutrophilia, which are consistent with bacterial meningitis.

A surgical procedure was considered to remove the damaged tissues. The patient was treated with heparin and fresh frozen plasma (FFP) and was placed on antimicrobial therapy. His electrolyte imbalance was corrected with fluids. Necrotic tissues were surgically removed. Although his DIC was resolved, he remained thrombocytopenic. Mr. Chowning was discharged from the hospital and was followed up as an outpatient.

PATIENT: ANGELINA CORTEZ

Study Questions A

1. *Clinical Symptoms*: Fever, fatigue, pallor, lethargy, weakness, petechiae, ecchymoses

    Background History: Bruised easily, decreased appetite, weight loss

2. CBC, electrolytes, glucose, BUN

4. a. Highly elevated WBC, decreased RBC, extremely low hemoglobin and hematocrit, extremely low platelet count. Blasts were seen on the peripheral blood smear. Differential count showed neutropenia (1 percent segmented neutrophils) and 66 percent blasts. Decreased RBC and low platelet count suggest that the patient is severely anemic and thrombocytopenic. The presence of immature cells in the peripheral blood indicates that these cells have grown out of control in the bone marrow and have "spilled over" into the peripheral system.

    b. At presentation, the patient showed pallor and appeared weak and lethargic. These clinical presentations are seen in individuals with low hemoglobin and a decreased number of red blood cells. Severe thrombocytopenia may be the cause of the petechiae and ecchymoses observed in this patient.

Study Questions B

1. a. The initial diagnosis of acute myeloid leukemia (AML) was made based on the presence of blasts on the peripheral smear. Neutropenia is present in most AML patients.

    b. Thrombocytopenia, anisocytosis, poikilocytosis, and anemia are usually present in AML. The myeloblasts present appeared to have monoblastic nuclei but a granulocytic cytoplasm. A diagnosis of AML-M4 is based on the presence of both granulocytic and monocytic precursors. Peripheral blood and bone marrow cell morphology, histochemical classification, cell surface marker differentiation, and cytogenetic evaluation are used to confirm the diagnosis.

    c. A comprehensive histochemical classification system dividing AML into several major subtypes was developed by the French-American-British (FAB) cooperative group. Special histochemical stains should be performed on bone marrow specimens of all children with acute leukemia to confirm their diagnosis. Immunophenotyping can also be helpful in distinguishing some FAB subtypes of AML. Testing for the presence of HLA-DR, which is expressed on 75 to 80 percent of AML but rarely on acute promyelocytic leukemia (APL), is also helpful.

2. Using monoclonal antibodies that determine cell surface antigens of AML cells is helpful in supporting the histologic diagnosis. Various lineage-specific monoclonal antibodies that detect antigens on AML cells are used in making a leukemia diagnosis in combination with a battery of lineage-specific T- and B-lymphocyte markers to help differentiate AML from ALL and other mixed-lineage or biphenotypic or biclonal leukemias. Cluster designations (CD) that are considered to be lineage-specific for AML include CD33, CD13, CD14, CDw41, CD15, CD11B, CD36 and antiglycophorin A.

3. Chromosomal analyses are important as diagnostic and prognostic markers in children with AML. Clonal chromosomal abnormalities can be identified in the blasts of about 75 percent of children with AML and have become useful in identifying the subtypes with specific characteristics. Diagnostic applications of molecular technology, such as probes, and other newer cytogenetic techniques, such as fluorescence in situ hybridization (FISH), have afforded detection of cryptic abnormalities that were not evident with standard cytogenetic banding studies. This is especially important when optimal therapy differs.

4. AML is the most common type of myeloid malignancy in children. With appropriate induction chemotherapy, 75 to 85 percent of children with AML can achieve a complete remission. A prognostic factor for AML in children that seems to be consistent is the white blood cell count at diagnosis. Children who have a WBC count greater than 100,000/mm^3 have a poor prognosis.

This patient was diagnosed with AML-M4e, which is associated with abnormalities of chromosome 16 and may be associated with an improved overall prognosis. She is within the age group that has the highest rate of remission and is more likely to have a relapse-free remission.

CASE SUMMARY

PATIENT: ANGELINA CORTEZ

The patient is a 13-year-old female who was seen at the clinic because of complaints of fever, fatigue, and decreased appetite for the past 2 to 2½ weeks. She also complained of easy bruising, especially on arms and legs. On physical examination, the patient showed pallor, was febrile, and appeared weak and lethargic. The patient also revealed petechiae over her mouth, ecchymoses, and signs of weight loss that had occurred over the last 6 months. The patient was diagnosed with acute myelomonocytic leukemia with dysplastic eosinophils (AML-M4e).

The patient was given 6 units of platelets and 250 mL of packed RBCs followed by 10 mg of Lasix IV. The patient became stabilized.

M4e is a variant of M4. In AML (M4e), both granulocytic and monocytic precursors are present. Each cell line constitutes 20 to 80 percent of nucleated bone marrow cells. M4e is closely associated with an abnormal chromosome 16, including either a deletion or an inversion of the long arm (16q). Patients with a 16q abnormality and bone marrow eosinophilia have a longer median survival than patients with typical M4. The nuclei of these eosinophils are abnormal in morphology, cytochemical reactivity, and ultrastructure. The nucleus is not segmented, and, unlike normal eosinophils, these cells stain positive with naphthol ASD, chloracetate esterase, and PAS.

The age of the patient at the time of diagnosis has an important impact on the duration of the survival. Excluding those diagnosed in the neonatal period, children diagnosed in the first 15 years of life have the highest rate of remission and are more likely to have a relapse-free remission. Also, an elevated white cell count greater than 30×10^9/L or a blast count greater than 15×10^9/L at diagnosis decreases the probability of remission and the length of remission. If the patient does not receive any treatment or chemotherapy for the disorder, the median survival will be about 6 weeks. About 3 percent will survive for about a year. About 1 percent will survive longer. With a combination of intense chemotherapy, transfusions, and antibiotics, there is a strong possibility of complete remission. In children, the remission rate is 90 percent.

ANSWERS TO LEARNING ACTIVITIES 1

PATIENT: MICHELLE CRAIG

Study Questions A

1. *Clinical Symptoms:* Dehydration, petechiae

   Background History: Vomiting, diarrhea

2. *CBC, *CMP, urinalysis, platelet count

   * = Tests that correlate with presenting symptoms

4. Yes. Increased WBC, neutrophils, BUN, glucose, and cholesterol; decreased RBC, Hgb, Hct, platelets, lymphocytes, and potassium; bacteria, red cells, and white cells in urine

5. a. Yes, the significantly decreased platelet count

   b. Dehydration, urinary tract infection, thrombocytopenia, inflammation

   c. Yes, the 10-day history of vomiting and diarrhea results in dehydration and also may contribute to a UTI. The decreased platelet count may account for the petechiae but the anemia is unexpected and should be investigated.

Study Questions B

1. Aplastic anemia, renal failure, hypothyroidism, acute and/or chronic blood loss, chloramphenicol, myelosuppressive drugs, hemoglobinopathies

iron deficiency, vitamin B_{12}/folic acid deficiency, anemia of chronic disease

2. Aplastic anemia; marrow infiltration due to leukemia, lymphoma, or carcinoma; radiation and myelosuppressive drugs; thiazide diuretics; chronic alcoholism; vitamin B_{12}/folic acid deficiency; viral infections; renal failure

3. Yes; viral infections

4. Arthralgia; arthritis; fever; skin rashes, especially facial; anemia, lymphopenia, thrombocytopenia; kidney damage; pleurisy; photosensitivity; alopecia; Raynaud's phenomenon; seizures; mouth or nose ulcers

5. The combination of anemia, lymphopenia, and thrombocytopenia is consistent with autoimmunity. On the following day, the extremely elevated sedimentation rate confirmed an inflammatory condition.

6. In an autoimmune thrombocytopenia, the antiplatelet antibodies destroy the viable platelets. The platelet transfusions simply gave the antibodies more platelets to destroy.

7. Most likely, it was an immune response that destroys platelets that caused the thrombocytopenia. Steroids are effective in reducing inflammation and suppressing the immune system.

8. Anemia; circulatory constriction in extremities; congestive heart failure; pericarditis; kidney damage; CNS problems; infections; joint, muscle, and bone damage

9. ANA titers, kidney function tests, CBC, inflammatory proteins

10. a. No

    b. Dehydration

11. On 1/29/94, the C-reactive protein was 22.8 mg/dL (normal range 0.0–1.8 mg/dL). CRP is another assay that detects generalized inflammation. Levels are increased with active SLE and decline when medications are used to reduce the inflammation. Ms. Craig's CRP indicates significant inflammation.

12. ANA   Positive, >1:320   (normal: negative)

    This is a screening test because it is positive in close to 100 percent of patients with active SLE. Ms. Craig has a significantly elevated ANA titer.

    ANA Pattern   Speckled and rim pattern

    This indicates that the interphase nucleus is staining with the fluorescent antibody while the chromosomes are not staining.

    C3 Complement   77.0   (normal range 83.0–177.0 mg/dL)

    Complement proteins mediate inflammation and are useful in evaluating kidney involvement and in monitoring the disease over time. The mildly decreased C3 complement indicates no renal involvement at this point.

Anti-DNA   Positive   (normal: negative)

Anti-DNA is an immunoglobulin that is specific against double-stranded DNA. It is highly specific for SLE and may be used as a measure of disease activity.

Extractable Nuclear Antibodies:

Anti-Sm   1:32

This is an antibody specific against Sm, a ribonucleoprotein found in the cell nucleus. It is also highly specific for SLE.

Anti-RNP   1:32

This is an antibody to ribonucleoprotein that is not particularly specific for SLE.

Anti-SS-A   Negative

Anti-SS-B   Negative

These two antibodies are specific against RNA proteins. Anti-SS-A is found in only 30 percent of SLE patients, and anti-SS-B is found in only 15 percent of SLE patients.

Each of these results indicates a diagnosis of SLE in Ms. Craig.

13.   a.   To rule out other causes of anemia

   b.   Normal results

   c.   Ms. Craig does not have an iron deficiency that is causing her anemia.

14.   A direct antiglobulin test (DAT) test would indicate whether Ms. Craig's anemia is due to an autoimmune hemolytic anemia. A negative result would indicate an anemia of chronic disease, whereas a positive result would indicate that the anemia is due to autoimmunity caused by the SLE.

15.   Most of the tests ordered were appropriate for a significantly ill patient with SLE. In retrospect, the hepatitis profile did not give information of significance for this patient, but it was ordered to rule out hepatitis as a cause of Ms. Craig's gastroenteritis.

ANSWERS TO LEARNING ACTIVITIES 2

PATIENT: MICHELLE CRAIG

Study Questions A

1.   *Clinical Symptoms:* Diarrhea, vomiting, urinary urgency and burning

Background History: SLE for approximately 2½ years

2. CBC, *urine culture and sensitivity for UTI, CMP, sedimentation rate, rheumatology profile

   * = Tests that correlate with presenting symptoms

   Actually, none of the laboratory tests were ordered to evaluate her nausea and vomiting, although the CMP would indicate dehydration if present. The tests ordered were to assess the status of her preexisting condition, SLE, to see if this might be contributing to her current situation.

4. Yes; RBC, Hgb, Hct, sedimentation rate, BUN, creatinine, total protein, albumin, A/G ratio, calcium, cholesterol, phosphorus

   In urine, clarity, protein, albumin, blood, nitrite, WBCs, RBCs

   In the rheumatology profile, ANA, ANA titer, C3 complement

5. a. No

   b. Ms. Craig's SLE and anemia have not worsened since her initial diagnoses, but her renal function is deteriorating.

6. The positive urine culture identified Ms. Craig's urinary tract infection. Since the diarrhea and vomiting are unrelated to SLE, renal function, and anemia, they are probably the result of food poisoning. Her office visit presented an opportunity to assess her overall condition and reevaluate the SLE.

7. The CBC of 8/7/96 shows a worsened anemia, with the RBC count dropping from 3.68 to 3.05 and the hematocrit dropping from 32 to 26. The platelet count is well within the normal range at this point.

Study Questions B

1. The rheumatology profile is essentially unchanged over the past 2½ years, and the sedimentation rate continues to show significant inflammation.

2. BUN and creatinine are the classic renal function tests on serum. The BUN is slightly elevated, and the creatinine is at the top of the reference range. Serum total protein and albumin are decreased, indicating a loss of protein through the glomerulus. The creatinine clearance evaluation is significantly decreased, and the 24-h urine protein reflects the loss of protein into urine.

3. A creatinine clearance test is a measure of the kidney's glomerular filtration rate (GFR). It assesses the kidney's ability to maintain the normal composition of body fluids. Clearance tests are used to detect mild to moderate diffuse glomerular damage. In Ms. Craig's case, autoimmune damage to the glomerulus that limits the renal excretion of many substances and allows proteins to be excreted into the urine has occurred.

4. A 24-h urine sample is collected in a container with no preservatives and refrigerated between samples. A blood sample is drawn at some point within the 24-h urine collection period. The patient should maintain an adequate urine flow of at least 2 mL/min. Caffeine, medications, and heavy exercise should be avoided during the collection period. A creatinine assay is then performed on both the urine and blood samples, and the results are calculated to obtain creatinine clearance.

5. Creatinine clearance = $\dfrac{\text{urine cr} \times \text{urine volume}}{\text{plasma cr collection in minutes}}$

    A correction for body surface area may be added by dividing the standard body surface area (1.73 m^2) by the patient's body surface area. This result is then multiplied by the result obtained from the previous calculation.

6. Calcium concentrations are closely tied to protein concentrations in the blood, since nearly half of the circulating calcium is bound to protein. When protein concentrations drop, the calcium levels drop as well. Phosphorus concentrations fluctuate in an inverse relationship to calcium concentrations, so when the calcium concentration drops, the phosphorus concentration rises in response. The calcium and phosphorus abnormalities seen are thus a reflection of the decreased total protein concentrations.

ANSWERS TO LEARNING ACTIVITIES 3

PATIENT: MICHELLE CRAIG

Study Questions A

1. *Clinical Symptoms:* Weak, shaky, no appetite, nausea

    Background History: A 4½-year history of SLE, a 2-year history of lupus nephritis, anemia

2. CMP, CBC, sedimentation rate, *urinalysis, CRP, rheumatology profile, ECG

    * = Tests that correlate with presenting symptoms

4. a. Elevated sedimentation rate, urinary protein, blood, ketones, red and white cells

    Positive ANA titer

    Decreased WBC count, RBC count, hemoglobin, and hematocrit

    b. Abnormal urine results, especially urinary protein

5. a. No

    b. Ms. Craig's systemic lupus erythematosis, lupus nephritis, and anemia are essentially unchanged from her last evaluation. This indicates that there must be other changes or conditions that account for the worsening symptoms.

    c. Anemia correlates with her presenting symptom of fatigue, but Ms. Craig has had long-standing anemia and the fatigue is of only 1 week's duration. The patient is likely to have a viral disease with nonspecific symptoms, and none of the laboratory results ordered at this point will give us specific information about a particular viral infection.

6. Yes. Symptoms of hyperthyroidism include fatigue, weakness, weight loss, nervousness, increased sweating, and heart palpitations, all of which Ms. Craig exhibits.

7. The decrease in the TSH result point to a diagnosis of primary hyperthyroidism, which indicates that the thyroid gland itself is overproducing the thyroid hormones. If this were a secondary condition, the TSH result would be increased, as the pituitary gland would be overproducing TSH, which in turn would stimulate the thyroid gland to release thyroid hormones without a need for them. The presence of thyroid antibodies on 8/11/98 is helpful in the diagnosis of Graves' disease.

8. Thyrotropin receptor antibodies (TSHR) are found in approximately 95 percent of patients with Graves' disease, and thyroperoxidase antibodies (TPO) are seen in almost 75 percent of these patients.

Study Questions B

1. Yes, it is common for hyperthyroid patients to become hypothyroid after RAI treatment as a result of overdestruction of the thyroid tissue. However, it is much easier to treat hypothyroidism than hyperthyroidism. The other option for treatment would have been thyroid surgery, but this treatment is also likely to produce hypothyroidism.

2. Yes. SLE, lupus nephritis, and Graves' disease are all autoimmune conditions. It is common for persons with one autoimmune condition to develop others, as this case points out.

3. There were no tests omitted that might be helpful in Ms. Craig's diagnoses.

4. Thyroid profiles are being performed at frequent intervals, but in light of the changes in Ms. Craig's symptoms and treatments, these tests seem appropriate. The need for both a liver profile and a hepatitis profile and for the CMV and EBV titers performed on 8/3/98 is questionable.

CASE SUMMARY

PATIENT: MICHELLE CRAIG

Diagnosis 1: Ms. Craig was admitted to the hospital as a result of dehydration from gastroenteritis. In the process of her evaluation, she was found to have a severely decreased platelet count and anemia. Numerous platelet transfusions did not significantly increase her count, implying an autoimmune reaction. Further studies showed evidence of inflammation and prompted definitive tests for SLE. Treatment with steroids provided prompt clinical improvement. All diagnostic test results indicated SLE with no additional organ involvement at this point. Patient should be followed carefully to identify any renal or joint complications that may develop.

The course of SLE is unpredictable and varies with the degree of organ involvement and inflammatory response. Ten-year survival rates are 85 to 95 percent with treatment. SLE is a chronic, lifelong disease, with alternating periods of relapse (flares) and remission. Flares occur 2 to 3 times each year on average.

Diagnosis 2: About 2½ years after Ms. Craig was diagnosed with SLE, lupus nephritis had developed. This diagnosis was made from a renal biopsy after abnormal laboratory test results suggested deteriorating renal function. The patient was placed on Cytoxan to treat the kidney damage and to augment treatment with steroid medications.

Diagnosis 3: Ms. Craig is seen 2 years after her lupus nephritis diagnosis with symptoms that prove to be caused by Graves' disease. The Graves' disease was treated successfully with propylthiouracil for approximately 16 months, but then Ms. Craig's worsening anemia prompted consideration of alternative therapies for hyperthyroidism. It was felt that the PTU was depressing her bone marrow and exacerbating the anemia associated with her SLE. Ms. Craig was given a radioactive iodine uptake evaluation, which showed that her thyroid gland was absorbing iodine at 100 percent. A therapeutic dose of radioactive iodine was given, which returned her thyroid hormone studies into the reference range. A common complication of radioactive iodine therapy is that the patient becomes hypothyroid as a result of excessive destruction of thyroid tissue by the radioactive iodine. Ms. Craig's laboratory results indicate that she developed hypothyroidism 3 months after her radioactive iodine therapy. Ms. Craig is currently being successfully treated with Synthroid to correct the hypothyroidism.

ANSWERS TO LEARNING ACTIVITIES

PATIENT: KENYA FIELDER

Study Questions A

1. *Clinical Symptoms:* Abdominal pain, shortness of breath

   Background History: Received 2 units of packed RBCs 40 years prior

2. *CBC, electrolytes, PT, APTT, UA; type and cross-match for 4 units of packed RBCs. The rest of the laboratory tests requested are pre-operative tests since the patient was scheduled for surgery.

   * = Tests that correlate with presenting symptoms

4. a. Hemoglobin and hematocrit are outside the normal acceptable range, as is red blood cell morphology.

    b. The lab findings confirm the initial diagnosis of anemia. Additional tests are necessary to evaluate the diagnosis of hereditary elliptocytosis.

Study Questions B

2. Initial blood bank test results:

Patient Cells with			Patient Serum with	
Anti-A	Anti-B	Anti-D	A$_1$ cells	B cells
0	0	3+	4+	4+

Patient's ABO/Rh: O Rh (D) pos

3. 3-cell antibody screen: Negative

    4-unit red blood cell compatibility test: 3 of 4 units compatible

    Compatibility test results with four O positive red blood cell units:

Unit Number	Immediate Spin Compatibility Test Result
12156	0
12157	0
12158	4+
12159	0

   a. Yes, there are incompatibilities detected. The most probable cause of the incompatibility result is incorrect ABO typing of either the patient or the donor.

      All tests were repeated, and the identical results were produced.

   b. A segment should be removed from the unit and an ABO forward type should be performed on the red blood cells.

      Unit 12158 test results:

      Unit cell with

Anti-A	Anti-B	Anti-D	Unit label: O positive
4+	0	3+	

   c. Unit 12158 is labeled as O positive; however, the unit is actually A positive. The unit has been mislabeled. The anti-A and/or anti-A,B of the O positive patient is reacting with the A positive red blood cells of the donor.

   d. There can be many reasons for the mislabeling of this unit. They can include the testing of the incorrect whole blood donation specimen, the misinterpretation of ABO tests, the incorrect recording of the test results, and the placing of an incorrect label on the unit bag during the labeling process.

A complete investigation will need to be completed in order to determine the actual reason for the mislabeling of this unit.

4. One more O positive red blood cell unit should be selected for the patient. When this was done, the compatibility test showed compatibility between the patient and the donor. The 4 units of red blood cells are now ready to be issued if needed by the patient.

5. Many technical, clerical, or procedural errors could have led to the mislabeling of the unit.

   The technologist was selecting products for compatibility testing. The laboratory had recently received a single box shipment of 15 O positive and 15 A positive units of red blood cells to replenish a low inventory. ABO confirmation testing was performed and documented, and the new units were placed on the available inventory shelf. Unit 12158 gave the incompatible test result. The area of the unit where segments are removed for ABO confirmation testing is bound with a rubber band. On closer investigation of the unit, it was discovered that the banded area of this unit contained both attached segments from the unit and unattached segments that had been detached from another unit in the shipment box and were now bound within the rubber band. When the two distinct segments were tested, it was discovered that the segment that was attached to the unit was A positive and that the unattached segment that was bound within the rubber band was O positive. During ABO confirmation testing, the incorrect segment was removed and tested. This gave a result that appeared to show a properly labeled O positive unit. During the compatibility testing, the correct segment was removed and tested. This gave a result that revealed the mislabeling of the unit.

6. The most common severe form of transfusion reaction is the acute hemolytic transfusion reaction. These reactions are usually caused by preformed antibodies that have the ability to activate the complement cascade and other biological cascades. The antibodies of the ABO system are most often implicated in these reactions.

CASE SUMMARY

PATIENT: KENYA FIELDER

This patient was fortunate that the error was detected in the laboratory. Had the technologist mistakenly removed one of the unattached segments that was bound by the segment rubber band, the unit would have tested as compatible in the laboratory. Because all testing would have appeared to be acceptable, the product would have been issued and transfused to the patient. It would then have been up to the person transfusing the unit to the patient to detect and treat the reaction.

The patient was able to receive all compatible red blood cell units following her surgery without incident.

The laboratory modified procedures to ensure that the segment being tested was attached to the unit prior to testing. The collection and processing center modified procedures to ensure the correct identity of a specimen used for ABO and other testing.

ANSWERS TO LEARNING ACTIVITIES

PATIENT: ALFRED GATES

Study Questions A

1. *Clinical Symptoms*: Chronic fatigue, fever, pain in his right groin

   Background History: Smoked two packs of cigarettes per day for 6 to 7 years, occasional alcohol consumption, no drug usage, history of coronary artery disease in family

2. *CBC, *tissue biopsy of lymph node in the right groin

   * = Tests that correlate with presenting symptoms

4. a. Elevated white blood cell count (40,000/μL) 40 $\times$ 10^9/L, decreased red blood cell count (3 million/mL), thrombocytopenia (platelet count of 9,000/μL) 9 $\times$ 10^9/L, anemia (hemoglobin of 6.4 g/dL and hematocrit of 18.1 percent)

   b. The peripheral blood smear showed a large number of what appeared as abnormal, cerebriform lymphocytic cells. Smudge cells were present in large numbers. The lymphocytes and all other abnormal cells possessed a vacuolated cytoplasm. The bone marrow showed several mast cells and reactive-appearing lymphocytes, and all stages of the lymphocytic development had vacuolated cytoplasm. Slight poikilocytosis with teardrop and burr cells were also observed. Schistocytes were present.

5. CT scan of the chest showed lymph node adenopathy, and CT scan of the abdomen showed splenomegaly.

6. Based on the biopsy of the lymph node taken from the groin, the initial diagnosis was peripheral T-cell lymphoma, unspecified. The staging is done by looking at the rest of the body to see what else is involved. In this case, the involvement of the bone marrow determines that the patient has stage IV disease.

7. Cytarabine is an antimetabolite that is used to treat leukemia and other types of cancer. Cytarabine interferes with the growth of cancer cells; how-

ever, it also affects normal body cells. Patients are warned about the complications and side effects, such as hair loss, that may develop as a result of treatment with cytarabine. Breast feeding is not recommended while receiving treatment. Cytarabine may also cause birth defects; therefore, female patients are warned against pregnancy during the course of therapy. Because chemotherapeutic agents cause immunosuppression, patients are warned about their susceptibility to infections. They are instructed not to have any immunizations without their physician's approval.

Study Questions B

1. *Candida tropicalis*

2. *Candida* species are members of the usual microbial flora found on the skin and mucous membranes. In most cases, they do not cause disease, but they are often found as opportunists when the immune defenses of the host are compromised. Patients with leukemia are usually infected with *Candida* species, usually *C. albicans* and *C. tropicalis*. These findings are consistent with Mr. Gates's diagnosis of T-cell lymphoma, as he has received chemotherapeutic and immunosuppressive drugs.

3. This finding indicates that Mr. Gates is at risk for more systemic infections as he continued to receive his treatments.

4. High-grade T-cell lymphomas such as this one represent less than 10 percent of the non-Hodgkin's malignancies. The severity of the infiltration is described using a classification system. This case is a stage IV. Stage IV is used to define a lymphoma that also involves some organ other than the lymph nodes or spleen, such as the lungs or bone marrow. This is a very severe dissemination of malignancy. Patients become susceptible to various bacterial infections and eventually succumb to these infections.

CASE SUMMARY

PATIENT: ALFRED GATES

The case study presented here is an example of a T-cell lymphoma. The patient is a 56-year-old white male who presented with lymphadenopathy. The patient had a history of smoking two packs of cigarettes per day for 6 to 7 years, ceasing in 1991. He reported occasional consumption of alcohol and no drug usage. The family history showed no evidence of malignancies; however, there was a history of family members expiring due to coronary artery disease.

The initial diagnosis was peripheral T-cell lymphoma, unspecified. A biopsy of the right groin lymph node was performed. A CT scan of the chest demonstrated lymph node adenopathy, and a CT scan of the abdomen showed splenomegaly. The patient's laboratory findings showed a thrombocytopenia and an anemia, with a hemoglobin of 6.4 g/dL and a hematocrit of 18.1%. His platelet count was 9000/μL. An average white count was approximately 40,000/μL, and the red count was 3 million.

A peripheral blood smear displayed a large number of abnormal, blast-looking cells. Smudge cells were also present in large numbers. These have prominent blue-staining nucleoli. There was slight poikilocytosis, with teardrop and burr cells. Schistocytes were also observed. The lymphocytes and abnormal cells possessed a vacuolated cytoplasm. The bone marrow showed several mast cells and reactive-appearing lymphocytes. All stages of lymphocytic development had a vacuolated cytoplasm. Bone marrow core biopsy stained with H & E is evaluated and shows clusters or sheets of atypical mononuclear cells; T-cell origin is determined with immunohistochemistry. Another way to support involvement is by getting T-cell receptor gene rearrangement studies performed on the bone marrow in conjunction with an abnormal morphology. The patient was then administered an antileukemic drug, cytarabine, which was later discontinued because of the formation of an abscess within the patient's groin region.

Several months later, the patient suffered a relapse, with small preauricular nodes, i.e., the area located in front of the ear. The biopsy was significant for recurrent lymphoma. He also had right inguinal lymph adenopathy, mediastinal lymphadenopathy (via chest CT), and splenomegaly (by abdominal CT). The patient was given chemotherapy, which was later deemed to be successful, following a biopsy of the bone marrow. No lymphoma was present at this time.

The following month, the patient received an autologous bone marrow transplant following chemotherapy with cyclophosphamide, an antineoplastic agent. The drug is also used as an immunosuppressant in organ transplantation. Subsequent to the transplant, the patient had a blood culture that was positive for *Candida tropicalis*. He was treated with amphotericin B.

Several weeks later, the patient was started on IL-3, which is a proven antitumor agent. One month later, the patent again suffered a relapse and all previous symptomatology returned. The patient showed substantial lymphadenopathy of the chest and neck. A CT scan of the head, however, was normal. Chemotherapy was then continued. In October of the same year, the patient's condition was complicated by a methicillin-resistant *Staphylococcus aureus* (MRSA) infection. It was treated with vancomycin.

During the next few months, the patient continued on chemotherapy and was given numerous platelet transfusions as well as packed red cells. This same course is presently being followed with the patient.

ANSWERS TO LEARNING ACTIVITIES

PATIENT: GUYA GING

Study Questions A

1. *Clinical Symptoms:* Fatigue, weakness, unexplained bruises, rectal bleeding, petechiae over mouth

   Background History: Hypothyroidism

2.   *CBC, *PT, *APTT, *glucose, BUN, *electrolytes, *liver profile

   *Type and cross-match 2 units

   *Blood cultures × 2

   * = Tests that correlate with presenting symptoms

4.   a. Yes. RBC count, hemoglobin, and hematocrit are decreased. Platelet count is decreased. Total bilirubin and LDH values are elevated.

   b. The decreased RBC, hemoglobin, and hematocrit suggest anemia, which may explain her feeling fatigued and weak. The unexplained bruises, rectal bleeding, and petechiae are associated with thrombocytopenia. The increased bilirubin and LDH levels suggest hemolysis.

5.   a. Red blood cell morphology: Moderate to many schistocytes.

   b. Yes. The compatibility test and antibody screen are negative. No alloantibodies are detected. The direct antiglobulin test is negative. Donor units cross-matched are compatible.

6.   Blood cultures are negative. PT and APTT are within normal reference ranges.

Study Questions B

1.   a. Thrombotic thrombocytopenic purpura (TTP)

   b. In TTP, platelet count is greatly decreased. Total bilirubin and LDH levels are increased, while PT and APTT are generally normal. Decreased haptoglobin and the presence of schistocytes, helmet cells, burr cells, polychromasia, reticulocytosis, and hematuria are indicators of TTP.

   c. Platelet transfusion is contraindicated in TTP because it only exacerbates the patient's condition.

2.   The fibrin clots in the microvasculature make it difficult for red blood cells to pass through; hence, they are sheared, resulting in RBC fragmentation. This manifestation is seen in peripheral blood smears as fragmented red blood cells or schistocytes.

3.   Plasmapheresis or plasma exchange and infusion of large quantities of plasma are currently recommended as the mode of treatment for TTP. In plasma exchange, immune complexes are removed from the blood. Steroids, splenectomy, antiplatelet drugs, and immunoglobulin are other options.

4.   Based on the laboratory and clinical findings, the patient was diagnosed with TTP. The clinical and laboratory findings in TTP, however, are also seen in other disorders, such as ITP, HUS, and HELLP syndrome. DIC may also present similar findings.

   For differential diagnosis, in TTP, patients usually present with fever, petechiae, and bleeding because of the low platelet count. Increased bilirubin and LDH, reticulocytosis, and the presence of schistocytes on the smear are indications of hemolysis. Anemia is present in these patients but is uncommon in ITP. Prothrombin time and APTT are usually normal in patients with TTP, while PT and APTT are increased in DIC. D-dimer is positive in DIC, and thrombin time is prolonged. Thrombocytopenia is also seen in patients with SLE, usually as a result of peripheral destruction of platelets by autoantibodies or immune complexes. In SLE, the direct antiglobulin test is positive. Leukopenia is also common in SLE.

TTP, which occurs frequently in pregnant women, should be differentiated from HUS and the HELLP syndrome. TTP, if it remains untreated can be hazardous for pregnant women and the newborn.

5. After 20 plasma exchanges of about 6 units of plasma per exchange, the platelet count gradually increased to normal ($200,000/\mu L$), and the LDH values returned to the normal reference range.

6. Ms. Ging's clinical presentations and laboratory findings correlated well with the clinical and laboratory indicators of TTP. The patient showed thrombocytopenia, anemia, elevated liver enzymes, and hematuria. However, her coagulation studies were normal. Her blood smears showed numerous schistocytes.

7. The patient showed good prognosis. After 20 TPE, the patient's LDH levels returned to within the normal reference range and platelet count stabilized at $200,000/\mu L$.

CASE SUMMARY

PATIENT: GUYA GING

The patient is a 35-year-old female who presented with complaints of fatigue for the past month. She also complained of easy bruising, especially on her arms and legs, and felt weak and feverish. She reported a 2-day history of bright red blood from her rectum. The patient also had a history of hypothyroidism. On physical examination, the patient showed pallor, was febrile, and appeared weak. The patient also revealed acute rectal bleeding, petechiae over her mouth, and ecchymoses on her arms and inner thighs. Her laboratory findings revealed thrombocytopenia, anemia, and elevated liver enzymes. She also showed hematuria. Blood smears showed numerous schistocytes.

The patient was transfused with 2 units of packed red blood cells and 8 units of platelets after she was admitted to the facility. Although her hemoglobin and hematocrit were stabilized, her platelet count remained unchanged. The diagnosis of thrombotic thrombocytopenic purpura was established based on the presence of blood in the urine, schistocytes, decreased hemoglobin, elevated LDH, and thrombocytopenia.

The patient underwent 20 plasma exchanges of about 6 units of plasma per exchange. Platelet transfusion is contraindicated because it worsens the situation by leading to additional platelet clumping and aggregation. The patient's LDH levels returned to within the normal reference range and her platelet count became stable at 200,000/μL. The patient was discharged after 17 days in the hospital.

ANSWERS TO LEARNING ACTIVITIES

PATIENT: JANUS GLASS

Study Questions A

1. *Clinical Symptoms:* Productive cough, hemoptysis, fatigue, shortness of breath, fever, weakness, bullous lesions in lungs

    Background History: Positive PPD, asbestos exposure, alcohol abuse, smoking, worked with insecticides

2. *CBC, *PT, *APTT, *glucose, *BUN, *electrolytes, *sputum direct smear and culture

    * = Tests that correlate with presenting symptoms

4. a. CBC results showed decreased hemoglobin and hematocrit. Coagulation studies were prolonged.

    b. Decreased hemoglobin and hematocrit values may indicate anemia or that the patient is bleeding. These results correlate with the patient's symptoms of hemoptysis, fatigue, weakness, and shortness of breath. The prolonged coagulation tests results correlate with these symptoms as well.

5. The patient presents symptoms of a lower respiratory tract infection. However, sputum cultures produced normal respiratory flora. The direct sputum smear indicated that an acceptable sample was collected and submitted for culture and that an infectious disease was in progress. These findings were suggestive of etiologic agents that were probably nonbacterial in origin. The history of positive PPD and the presence of bullous lesions in the apical region of his lungs should be further investigated.

6. Mr. Glass's history of alcohol abuse, smoking, and exposure to asbestos and harmful chemicals that may have been present in insecticides may be considered as risk factors for respiratory illnesses. The positive PPD indicated past exposure to *Mycobacterium tuberculosis*.

7. Mr. Glass presented a lower respiratory tract infection. However, routine culture of respiratory secretions failed to yield a bacterial source, directing the clinician to investigate and examine other types of respiratory samples, such as bronchial washings. Mr. Glass's medical and work history were risk factors that have been associated with infectious agents such as *M. tuberculosis* and fungi. These agents have been encountered in immune-suppressed or immunocompromised individuals.

Study Questions B

1. Bronchial washings for fungal cultures produced growth that was identified as *Histoplasma capsulatum var capsulatum*. Mycobacterial cultures remained pending. The bone marrow studies showed aggregates of lymphohistiocytes that contained intracellular organisms consistent with *H. capsulatum*. Several days after the bone marrow aspirate was obtained, fungal cultures grew what was identified as *H. capsulatum*. Similar results were obtained from the blood cultures.

2. *H. capsulatum* is found primarily in the environment, especially in soil that is enriched with nitrogen. The organisms are acquired by inhaling the microconidia. Therefore, the lungs become the primary site of infection. Although most individuals are asymptomatic, bronchial irritation and pneumonitis may occur, and the host may experience a flulike syndrome. The organisms are readily engulfed by local histiocytes but are able to multiply intracellularly. In immune-competent individuals, the organisms are cleared by the reticuloendothelial system. However, in immune-suppressed and immunocompromised hosts, such as Mr. Glass, the infection may manifest as a respiratory illness, but may also disseminate hematogenously. Given Mr. Glass's risk factors, he was highly susceptible to an opportunist such as *H. capsulatum*.

3. Mr. Glass continued to receive packed RBCs to stabilize his hemoglobin and hematocrit. However, his WBC and platelet counts remained low and drastically decreased. He was placed on amphotericin B, an antifungal agent, but did not respond to therapy. On 4/7, 24-h incubation results of blood cultures showed gram-negative rods, later identified as *Pseudomonas aeruginosa*. After 4/7, Mr. Glass continued to deteriorate. His coagulation studies showed signs of disseminated intravascular coagulation. The patient expired.

CASE SUMMARY

PATIENT: JANUS GLASS

A 49-year-old white male reported to a clinic for a follow-up for bacterial pneumonia. The patient complained of coughing up blood, very green sputum, weakness, fatigue, and shortness of breath. On admission, his chest X-ray showed that he had chronic bullous lesions in the lungs, especially in the apical region. The patient had a history of positive PPD and asbestos exposure. He worked with insecticides on a farm. The patient told the doctor of a drinking problem and also said that he smoked 3 to 4 packages of tobacco products a week. The patient denied night sweats or chills but had experienced slight weight loss.

A bronchoscopy was performed. The initial diagnosis was *Mycobacterium tuberculosis*.

Laboratory results showed decreased hemoglobin and hematocrit and prolonged coagulation studies. The patient received a total of 8 units of packed RBCs and fresh frozen plasma. The patient also developed a temperature of 101.7°F. His posttransfusion CBC brought his hematocrit to 30 percent and his hemoglobin to 10 g/dL. However, the patient's WBC dropped from $6.7 \times 10^9/L$ to $3.0 \times 10^9/L$. Transfusion of 2 units of packed RBCs per day maintained his hemoglobin at 11 g/dL. There was a continued low white count in spite of the repeated temperature spikes.

A second chest x-ray showed an infiltrate attributed to either mucus plugs or pleural effusion. Bronchoscopy and blood cultures using the Dupont Isolator system were obtained. A bone marrow tap was also performed. The bone marrow was cultured for AFB, fungus, and bacteria and sent for histologic studies. At this time, the patient's WBC was $1.8 \times 10^9/L$ and platelets were $21,000/\mu L$. His hemoglobin and hematocrit remained stable.

The bone marrow studies revealed lymphohistiocytic aggregates with intracellular organisms. Seven days after the bone marrow was obtained, the fungal culture grew white, cottony colonies on Sabouraud dextrose agar at room temperature. Blood cultures from the Isolator grew the same. At 37°C, the fungus demonstrated the yeast form on brain-heart infusion blood agar. The isolate was identified as *Histoplasma capsulatum*.

The patient did not respond to therapy with amphotericin B. He developed bacterial septicemia and disseminated intravascular coagulation. The patient expired 6 weeks from the day of admission.

ANSWERS TO LEARNING ACTIVITIES

PATIENT: ROBERTO GUERERO

Study Questions A

1. *Clinical Symptoms*: Fever, leg pains, soft tissue swelling

   Background History: Laënnec's cirrhosis, GI bleeding, alcohol abuse, smoking

2. *CBC, *urinalysis, *culture of exudates and blood, *PT, *APTT, *glucose, *BUN, *electrolytes

   * – Tests that correlate with presenting symptoms

4. Staphylococcal and streptococcal cellulitis manifest as a soft tissue infection characterized by blisterlike lesions (bullae) similar to those seen on this patient. Other organisms that should be considered include *Aeromonas hydrophila* and *Vibrio vulnificus*.

5. The patient's hemoglobin and hematocrit were slightly decreased. His platelet count was also decreased. Coagulation studies were increased. Chemistry results were unremarkable.

Study Questions B

2. These parameters are indicators of impending disseminated intravascular coagulation.

3. Liver disease such as cirrhosis of the liver is a major risk factor. The patient also had a history of alcoholism.

4. *Aeromonas hydrophila* was isolated.

CASE SUMMARY

PATIENT: ROBERTO GUERERO

This patient was a 52-year-old Latin American male who was admitted through the Emergency Department and complained of bilateral leg pains. The pain started with his right lower calf and increased in intensity and was accompanied by swelling within hours of onset. The patient was febrile and reported chills but denied vomiting or diarrhea.

On admission, the patient was alert and oriented. His lungs were clear, and his heart rate was regular. He had a temperature of 101°F. His abdomen was soft and slightly protuberant, but there were no masses and no hepatomegaly or splenomegaly. Chest x-ray showed no effusion. A surgical scar from a portacaval shunt put in place several years ago was evident. The left lower extremity showed rash and tissue swelling.

Fifteen days prior to admission, the patient had undergone an upper GI endoscopy. The results showed duodenitis, but there was no deformity, edema, or any evidence of ulcer. The patient's previous history included Laënnec's cirrhosis, gastritis, and upper GI bleeding with several blood transfusions. Of note, a year previously, he had been treated for cellulitis in the left leg. The patient had drunk three cases of beer per week for the past 10 years and smoked heavily.

At the time of admission, the laboratory tests showed decreased hemoglobin and hematocrit values; the platelet count was also markedly decreased. On the other hand, prothrombin time (PT) and activated partial thromboplastin time (APTT) were greatly elevated. The admitting diagnosis was cellulitis of the legs, most probably due to *Staphylococcus* sp. or *Streptococcus* sp. Initial therapy with oxacillin was started.

The patient deteriorated rapidly within a few hours of his admission. The blisters developed into large bullae that progressed from his lower extremities to his trunk. Therapy was changed to multiple broad-spectrum antimicrobics, and treatment for a presumed diagnosis of disseminated intravascular coagulation associated with septic shock was also initiated. The patient was placed on a mechanical ventilator, and attempts were made to improve his blood pressure. However, he remained unresponsive to therapy and expired within several hours of his admission.

ANSWERS TO LEARNING ACTIVITIES

PATIENT: MEI LIN

Study Questions A

1. *Clinical Symptoms:* Uterine contractions; pregnant, in labor at full term

   Background History: One previous pregnancy 3 years ago; live birth. No prenatal records in this hospital.

   No history of transfusion. No medications. Latest visit to the other hospital was 3 months prior to delivery.

2. CBC, electrolytes, glucose, BUN, urinalysis. The laboratory tests requested on this patient are routine tests for admission.

4. All laboratory test results at the time of admission were within the reference range.

Study Questions B

2. a. Initial blood bank test results:

Patient Cells with				Patient Serum with	
Anti-A	Anti-B	Anti-D	Weak D	A_1 cells	B cells
0	0	3+	0	4+	4+

   ABO/Rh: A negative (weak D negative)

   b. **Antibody screen:** Positive (AHG phase only)

   Antibody identification: Anti-D

   Test for fetomaternal hemorrhage (FMH): Positive (Rosette screening test)

   The patient is D negative and the child is D positive; therefore, there is a risk that the patient will form anti-D if any amount of fetomaternal hemorrhage (FMH) occurred during the delivery.

   The patient has anti-D present in her serum. Not enough information is provided to determine if the patient is a candidate for RhIG.

   If this anti-D is due to prior immune stimulation of antibody production from a previous pregnancy or transfusion, then the patient would not be a candidate for RhIG. If this anti-D is due to previous administration of RhIG, then the patient would be a candidate for RhIG.

3. a. Tests to be performed on the child are

   ABO (forward type only), Rh (D), weak D testing if initially D negative, direct antiglobulin test (DAT), eluate from red blood cells if DAT is positive and clinical circumstances warrant, identification of antibody in eluate, hemoglobin/hematocrit, total bilirubin

Tests to be performed on the patient are ABO, Rh (D), weak D testing if initially D negative, antibody screen, antibody identification, if applicable

For FMH if patient is D negative and child is D positive

b. The child is O positive; therefore, there is no risk for ABO-HDN.

The mother of the child has anti-D in her serum, but since this antibody is due to a previous administration of RhIG, the child is not at risk for Rh-HDN.

The mother of the child has no other clinically significant antibodies in her serum; therefore, the child is not at risk for HDN caused by other clinically significant antibodies.

The hemoglobin/hematocrit and total bilirubin levels for the child are within the normal ranges. The positive DAT and presence of anti-D in the eluate of the child are due to the administration of RhIG to the mother of the child and do not appear to be causing any clinical problems for the child.

4. Consult the hospital where the patient was seen previously. Inquire about patient test results and transfusion history.

5. Results from consultation with the hospital where the patient was seen previously:

ABO/Rh: A negative (weak D negative)

Antibody screen: Negative

Transfusion history: Patient received one 300-μg dose of RhIG 3 months ago.

Since the patient has anti-D due to a previous administration of RhIG, the patient is a candidate for RhIG.

6. a. Since the rosette screening test for FMH is positive, more than one dose of RhIG may be needed for the patient.

The Kleihauer-Betke (acid elution) test will quantify the size of the FMH and indicate how many doses of RhIG are to be given to the patient.

Kleihauer-Betke (acid elution) test results:

20 fetal cells are counted within 2000 adult cells.

Kleihauer-Betke result: 20/2000 = 0.01 or 1.0 percent.

Volume of fetal bleed: 1.0×50 mL = 50 mL.

Number of doses of RhIG needed: 50 mL/30 mL per dose = 1.7 doses.

This calculation rounds up to 3 doses of RhIG of 300 μg each.

b. The risk of this patient in producing immune-stimulated anti-D following exposure to the D antigen is as follows:

One dose of RhIG given at 28 weeks' gestation and one dose of RhIG given <72 h following the delivery of the child: 0.1 percent

c. One dose of RhIG given <72 h following the delivery of the child: 1.0 percent

d. No doses of RhIG given during the pregnancy: 13.0 percent

CASE SUMMARY

PATIENT: MEI LIN

The patient met all three criteria to be a candidate for RhIG. The patient's antibody screen demonstrated the presence of anti-D. The origin of the anti-D as a result of previous administration of RhIG was confirmed by contacting the hospital where the patient was seen previously. The results of the rosette screening test and the Kleihauer-Betke (acid elution) test revealed the need for additional doses of RhIG for the patient. A total of three doses of RhIG are administered to the patient to prevent the formation of immune anti-D following the delivery of a D antigen–positive child. Because the patient received a dose of RhIG at 28 weeks' gestation and the calculated dose of RhIG <72 h after the delivery of a D antigen–positive child, the patient now has a 0.1 percent risk of forming immune anti-D.

The child of the patient is group O and at no risk for ABO-HDN. The antibody screen and medical history of the patient revealed only the presence of anti-D due to the previous administration of RhIG in the serum of the patient. These results show that the child has no risk for D-HDN or other-HDN. The test results obtained from the child's specimen show that the child is not experiencing any clinical problems.

ANSWERS TO LEARNING ACTIVITIES

PATIENT: MINH SANG NGO

Study Questions A

1. *Clinical Symptoms:* Bruises, fatigue, fever, necrotic lesion

Background History: Chronic fatigue, pallor, fever, easy bruising. Previously diagnosed with malignancy and received chemotherapy. Treatment failed. Received autologous bone marrow transplant.

2. *CBC, *glucose, *BUN, *electrolytes; *blood cultures; *bacterial, *fungal, and *AFB cultures of biopsied lesion

   * = Tests that correlate with presenting symptoms

4. WBC, RBC, hemoglobin, hematocrit, platelet count

5. The test results listed in question 4 are all below the acceptable reference ranges. Decreased hemoglobin, hematocrit, and RBC count suggest anemia and account for Mr. Ngo's fatigue and pallor. His easy bruising is due to the low platelet count.

6. a. Acute myeloid leukemia

   b. Evaluation of laboratory test results provided the presumptive diagnosis based on the morphology of the cells seen on peripheral blood and bone marrow aspirates. The patient showed extreme anemia, and the presence of immature neutrophilic precursors was evident on the smears. Auer rods were present; Type I and Type II myeloid blasts with greater than 10 percent of the myeloid cells showed maturation.

   The bone marrow was markedly hypocellular (<10 percent), with no aggregates, infiltrates, granulomas, or fibrosis.

   c. Cytogenetic study and monoclonal antibodies help determine the type or classification of leukemia or malignancy the patient has. It also aids the physician in selecting appropriate therapy and in monitoring the efficacy of treatment.

7. The early chromosomal analysis report showed 16 percent of the cells with translocations and deletions that are associated with AML-M2; the more recent analysis showed 80 percent of the cells with the same translocations and deletions, indicating that the disease has worsened.

Study Questions B

1. a. In spite of the aggressive chemotherapy, the patient showed signs of relapse. An autologous bone marrow transplant was performed. An autologous bone marrow transplant is done when a compatible donor cannot be found. In this procedure, a certain amount of the patient's marrow is removed while the patient is in complete remission. The marrow is treated with monoclonal antibodies or 4-hydroxycyclophosphamide to remove any residual leukemic cells and then cryopreserved. The patient receives the marrow back when all traces of leukemic cells are gone.

   Peripheral stem cells can also be used to renew hematopoiesis in the marrow after intensive chemotherapy. Hematopoietic growth factor

(HGF) has also been used to stimulate leukemic cells to proliferate to a specific stage at which these cells become more susceptible to specific growth-phase cytotoxic drugs.

b. It seemed that the autologous bone marrow transplant on this patient has failed; hence, there are very limited options left and the patient's prognosis is poor. An allogenic bone marrow transplant is unlikely because of the patient's ethnicity; a compatible donor is highly unlikely to be found. Chemotherapy and supportive transfusions are options that the physician may discuss with the child's parents.

2. a. Cultures of the skin lesions for bacterial and fungal agents were negative.

c. The epithelial disorder that appeared 5 days posttransplantation and was suspected to have been due to an infectious agent was consistent with graft-versus-host disease (GVHD). The negative cultures confirmed this diagnosis.

3. a. GVHD is a frequent complication of bone marrow transplant. It occurs when the donor's T lymphocytes recognize the patient as a new and foreign host. The T lymphocytes then begin to attack the new host's organs and tissues, including the skin, liver, and gastrointestinal tract. T lymphocytes are also able to recognize the differences in human leukocyte antigen genetic markers.

b. Although extensive typing of the donor and recipient is performed to match the genetic markers as closely as possible, differences will still occur unless the patient and the donor are identical twins. Approximately 50 percent of patients who receive mismatched transplants from family members or unrelated donor transplants develop GVHD. In most cases, it is mild; however, it can be a severe life-threatening complication. Patients with GVHD become more susceptible to infections.

c. The major organs and tissues affected by GVHD are the skin, liver, and gastrointestinal tract. The first signs of GVHD appear on the skin. Patients develop a skin rash that appears on the hands, feet, and face. The rash then spreads to other parts of the body, such as the scalp, upper chest, back, and abdomen. Some patients may develop blisters, an indication of severe GVHD. Involvement of the gastrointestinal tract is indicated by diarrhea and abdominal cramps. The linings of the small intestines, in particular, are primarily affected. The patient experiences severe cramping when the intestinal mucosal membranes are lost and the peristaltic movement of the small intestine becomes irregular. Jaundice is an indication that the liver is affected.

d. Numerous approaches have been used to decrease the occurrence or minimize the risk for GVHD. T-cell depletion or elutriation is a process wherein the lymphocytes from the donor bone marrow are removed by centrifugation. A certain amount of lymphocytes may remain, but these lymphocytes are needed for engraftment. The T-cell-depleted marrow graft is populated primarily with the stem cells needed to repopulate the bone marrow.

Drugs to prevent graft rejection are also used. Cyclosporine is an immunosuppressive drug given to bone marrow transplant recipients to suppress the ability of the donor's T cells to launch an attack against the recipient's organs. Methotrexate is another drug that is used in combination with cyclosporine. Patients who develop GVHD are usually treated with steroids.

CASE SUMMARY

PATIENT: MINH SANG NGO

The patient was a 7-year-old male child who presented with an epithelial disorder 5 days after a bone marrow transplant. Six months prior, the child was diagnosed with of acute myeloid leukemia (AML) based on the morphology of cells seen on peripheral blood and bone marrow aspirates. The patient showed extreme anemia, and the presence of immature neutrophilic precursors and Auer rods was evident on the smears. Cytogenetic study, cytochemical stains, and flow cytometry using monoclonal antibodies provided the FAB classification of AML-M2.

The patient received an aggressive regimen of chemotherapy. However, the child showed signs of relapse, and an autologous bone marrow transplant was performed, but the autologous transplant also failed. The epithelial disorder that appeared 5 days posttransplantation, characterized by purpura, especially in the legs, and histologically by exudation of neutrophils and fibrin around the dermal venules, was consistent with graft-versus-host disease, and the negative cultures for bacterial or fungal agents ruled out infection.

An allogenic bone marrow transplant was an unlikely option because of Mr. Ngo's ethnicity; a compatible donor was highly unlikely to be found. The patient's prognosis was poor. His functional immune leukocytes and immune response would continue to decline, making him more susceptible to infections, particularly bacteremia. Bacterial sepsis in leukemic patients is usually caused by *Staphylococcus aureus*, *Escherichia coli*, *Klebsiella pneumoniae*, or *Pseudomonas aeruginosa* and is a common cause of mortality among these patients.

Chemotherapy and supportive transfusions were options that the physician discussed with the child's parents.

PATIENT: GEORGE PITT

Study Questions A

1. *Clinical Symptoms:* Unexplained dull pain on his right side, fever, nausea

   Background History: Previous hospitalization and surgery to remove swallowed toothpick. Received 2 units of packed red blood cells.

2. *CBC, electrolytes, PT, APTT

   * = Tests that correlate with presenting symptoms

4. a. Mr. Pitt's hemoglobin and hematocrit are decreased. White blood cell count is increased. There is a shift to the left with the high number of bands and neutrophil count in the differential. Sodium and potassium are slightly decreased.

   b. The elevated white count with a shift to the left usually indicates the presence of a bacterial infection. The decreased hemoglobin and hematocrit show that the patient is slightly anemic. There is a slight electrolyte imbalance, probably due to minor dehydration from vomiting and diarrhea.

5. Yes. All pretransfusion testing results are normal, and there is no unusual history that would prevent these products from being issued for transfusion.

Study Questions B

2. a. A bacterial infection could be the cause of the elevated temperature. A postsurgical bleed could be the cause of the low hemoglobin/hematocrit. A transfusion reaction could be the cause of all of these test results.

   b. All laboratory tests requested; CBC, bilirubin, and blood cultures.

3. a. A posttransfusion specimen along with all transfusion-related items are to be sent to the blood bank laboratory. Since the transfusions took place 3 days ago, the red blood cell product bags and the infusing solutions have been discarded. The transfusion documents that were attached to the products and the posttransfusion specimen are sent to the blood bank laboratory.

   b. The blood bank must perform a clerical check on all paper and computer records related to the transfusion. A plasma hemolysis check and a direct antiglobulin test (DAT) must also be performed on the posttransfusion specimen.

4. A DAT should be performed on the pretransfusion specimen to use as a comparison with the DAT on the posttransfusion specimen.

An antibody identification on the eluate should be performed to detect the presence of an alloantibody or autoimmune antibody.

5. a. Retrieve the pretransfusion specimen and repeat all pretransfusion testing on both the pretransfusion specimen and the posttransfusion specimen.

Antibody enhancement techniques are used on the pretransfusion specimen to detect the presence of any allo- or autoantibody; in this case, there was no antibody detected on the pretransfusion sample. Phenotyping the red blood cell units is useful to detect Jk^a antigen in the transfused red blood cells; phenotyping of the 2 units transfused to this patient revealed that both units were positive for the Jk^a antigen.

b. Based on the symptoms, the timing, and the test results, this patient experienced a delayed hemolytic transfusion reaction caused by the antibody most commonly associated with this kind of reaction, anti-Jk^a. Unlike acute hemolytic transfusion reactions, where the symptoms appear within minutes, delayed transfusion reactions occur several days posttransfusion. In this patient, the reaction occurred within days following transfusion and is therefore a delayed one. This reaction is noninfectious because it is not the result of the transfusion of a bacterial, viral, or other agent.

c. Other than not transfusing the patient, no test would have prevented this transfusion reaction. The clinical signs indicated that the patient required the transfusion.

d. Keep a history of this antibody in the medical records of this patient at the hospital. Transfuse only red blood cell products that are negative for the Jk^a antigen. To prevent this transfusion reaction from occurring several years from now at another facility, provide the patient with an antibody identification card that lists the antibody. This card is to be presented on admission to any hospital.

CASE SUMMARY

PATIENT: GEORGE PITT

This patient produced anti-Jk^a from his red blood cell transfusion 3 years ago. No clinical reactions were seen at that time. In the following years, the serum titer of the antibody dropped below the level detectable on the pretransfusion antibody screen. All pretransfusion tests were performed correctly by the laboratory, and the 2 units of red blood cells were properly issued for transfusion.

Following the transfusion of the 2 Jk^a positive red blood cell units, the serum antibody titer rose and the antibodies coated and cleared the transfused cells. A mild fever occurred, and the posttransfusion hemoglobin/hematocrit did not rise to the expected levels.

Laboratory investigation of the transfusion reaction revealed the presence of the antibody in the posttransfusion specimen only. Because of this new antibody identification in the patient, all future red blood cell transfusions must be negative for the Jk^a antigen, even if the antibody screen is negative. This antibody identification must be a permanent part of the laboratory record of the patient. The patient may also be issued an antibody identification card in case of future transfusions at another medical facility.

ANSWERS TO LEARNING ACTIVITIES

PATIENT: WALTER REEVE

Study Questions A

1. *Clinical Symptoms:* Light-headed, weak, bruises easily

   Background History: The patient fell and suffered some bruises. History of small hematomas.

2. *Hemoglobin, *hematocrit, *bleeding time, *PT, *APTT

   * = Tests that correlate with presenting symptoms

4. a. Yes, APTT and bleeding time

   b. A coagulopathy

Study Questions B

2. All laboratory test results are normal except for the prolonged APTT result. A large hematoma was developed in a major joint area of the body following a short fall. An x-ray can be performed to reveal any bone damage. Coagulation factor assays can be performed to reveal any coagulation factor deficiencies.

3. Coagulation factors VIII and IX assays were performed. Factor VIII level is well below normal. The patient can be diagnosed with mild hemophilia A.

4. Factor VIII concentrate is the best product to give the patient to treat his hemophilia A. It provides a large amount of factor VIII in a small volume. Just 50 mL of product can contain thousands of units of factor VIII.

   Cryoprecipitate made from fresh frozen plasma is an alternative product that can be given to the patient. This product contains a concentrated amount of factor VIII in a relatively small volume. At least 80 units of factor VIII are found in each 15-mL bag.

Fresh frozen plasma is a product that contains a moderate amount of factor VIII in a large volume. One unit of factor VIII is found in each milliliter of product; therefore, a 225-mL bag of fresh frozen plasma will contain 225 units of factor VIII. The large volume that would be required to treat the patient does not make this a desirable product.

5. **Patient weight:** 132 lb (60 kg)

   Patient blood volume: 60 kg × 70 mL/kg = 4200 mL

   Patient plasma volume: 4200 mL × (1.0 Hct – 0.42 Hct) = 2436 mL

   Units of factor VIII required: 2436 mL × (0.50 unit/mL – 0.06 unit/mL) = 1072 units

6. Number of bags of cryoprecipitate required: 1072 units/80 units per bag = 13–14 bags.

7. No. ABO/Rh antigens and antibodies are not present in factor VIII concentrate.

   Cryoprecipitate contains small amounts of ABO antibodies. This product does not need compatibility testing with the patient prior to issue. An ABO/Rh type is the only test result needed prior to product selection. The previous ABO/Rh record on the patient eliminates the need for a new specimen.

8. A conservative approach would be to prepare plasma products that are compatible with the red blood cells of the patient. In this case, products with the ABO/Rh of A positive, A negative, AB positive, or AB negative would be compatible with the patient.

   Since cryoprecipitate products contain very little plasma, it may be acceptable to administer this product without considering the ABO/Rh compatibility.

   The Rh type of cryoprecipitate is not required to be on the product label. Most products do, however, come labeled with the complete ABO/Rh type.

9. The minimum amount of factor VIII required to be in each unit of cryoprecipitate is 80 units per bag, or 80 units times the number of bags in a pooled product.

   Thus, 14 bags of cryoprecipitate must contain 80 units of factor VIII per bag × 14 bags, or 1120 total units of factor VIII in the pooled product.

CASE SUMMARY

PATIENT: WALTER REEVE

This patient presented with a hematoma at the site of a major bone joint and a history of medically untreated hematomas at other bone joints. The laboratory results did not reveal an anemia, but they revealed a coagulation factor deficiency. The factor VIII deficiency, based on the factor assay, shows that the patient has mild hemophilia A (6 to 30 percent factor activity). Patients with mild hemophilia A can usually be managed without factor replacement therapy; however, because this patient has suffered a recent injury, the patient's physician ordered factor replacement therapy.

The calculation of the amount of factor needed is dependent on the weight, blood volume, and plasma volume of the patient. A standard formula is used to calculate the final amount of product needed for replacement therapy in factor I, VIII, and IX deficiencies.

The final requirement of 1072 units of factor VIII can best be delivered to the patient in the form of factor VIII concentrate. If this product is not available, then pooled cryoprecipitate can be given as an alternative.

The half-life of factor VIII is 12 h. Initial extravascular equilibration of newly infused factor VIII reduces the half-life to 4 h. To maintain a certain hemostatic level of factor, repeat infusions of product are given at 8- to 12-h intervals.

ANSWERS TO LEARNING ACTIVITIES

PATIENT: PAUL L. RICHMOND

Study Questions A

1. *Clinical Symptoms:* Pain on exertion and, later, at rest, nausea

    Background History: Increased lipids, previous PCTA, smoker, family history

2. CBC, UA, CMP, *cardiac profile, *lipid profile, *ABG

    * = Tests that correlate with presenting symptoms

4. a. WBC, Hct, Hgb, AST, total CK, CK-MB, troponin I, pH, Pco_2, Po_2, % Hgb saturation

    b. AST, total CK, CK-MB, troponin I

    c. Each of these results indicates significantly increased concentrations, which is consistent with myocardial injury.

    d. Acute myocardial infarction

5. Yes, all of Mr. Richmond's symptoms are indicative of AMI. Other symptoms that might be expected are left arm pain, shortness of breath, decreased blood pressure, sweating, and vomiting.

6. Hyperlipidemia, smoking, overweight, history of PTCA, and family history of coronary artery disease

7. Respiratory acidosis

8. Yes; reduced blood flow to the lungs prevents the release of CO_2, leading to acidosis.

Study Questions B

1. It takes at least 4 to 10 h from the onset of chest pain before CK-MB activities increase to significant levels in the blood. Peak levels occur within the first 24 h, and serum activities usually return to baseline levels within 2 to 3 days.

2. Yes

3. After an AMI, the troponin I increases above the reference range between 3 and 8 h after the onset of chest pain, peaks at 12 to 24 h, and returns to within reference limits after 5 to 10 days, depending on AMI size.

4. Yes

5. The myoglobin concentration was within reference limits on admission. Since myoglobin returns to a normal level within 10 to 12 h of the onset of pain and Mr. Richmond began having pain at least 48 h prior to admission, there is no indication for additional myoglobin assays.

6. This patient presented too late; these treatments must be initiated within 6 h of the onset of pain.

7. A baseline lipid profile is needed for future therapy decisions and risk stratification of this patient. Lipid concentrations may drop significantly after an AMI and will not return to pre-AMI concentrations for up to 2 months.

8. It is common for WBC counts to be elevated with AMI as a result of stress.

9. Mr. Richmond is somewhat anemic, but this is probably unrelated to this event. The anemia should be corrected, and this would be a part of a sensible diet and exercise program.

CASE SUMMARY

PATIENT: PAUL L. RICHMOND

This 63-year-old white male was seen in the ED with a 2-day history of chest and back pain. It was not accompanied by shortness of breath or vomiting, but the patient was nauseated. The patient stated that the pain occurred with activity and that it would take 1 to 2 h of rest for the pain to subside once it had occurred. Laboratory and ECG data indicated an acute myocardial infarction. The patient was admitted to the CCU for monitoring and evaluation by cardiology. A cardiac catheterization revealed stenosis in two coronary arteries; this was corrected with percutaneous transluminal coronary angioplasty 2 days later. The patient had an uneventful course after the procedure and was discharged with instructions for diet and exercise.

Mr. Richmond's coronary artery stenosis has been corrected by the PTCA procedure, but the underlying processes that led to the development of the stenosis remain. He should be advised to lose weight, initiate a regular exercise program, continue to take lipid-reducing medications while adhering to a low-fat diet, and take any other medications that would preserve cardiac functions. The myocardial damage caused by the AMI is irreversible, but considering the patient's age and good general health his condition should not further deteriorate. If these instructions are followed, Mr. Richmond should have a good prognosis.

ANSWERS TO LEARNING ACTIVITIES

PATIENT: WALTER ROBERTS

Study Questions A

1. *Clinical Symptoms:* Severe nausea, vomiting, scleral icterus

   Background History: Sudden onset of symptoms in an apparently healthy male, acetaminophen/alcohol combination

2. CBC, *urinalysis, *CMP, *PT, APPT

   * = Tests that correlate with presenting symptoms

4. a. BUN, creatinine, creatinine clearance, presence of albumin and casts in urine

   b. Total bilirubin, ALP, AST, ALT, PT, presence of bile and positive ictotest in urine

   c. Yes; liver enzymes, AST, ALT, BUN and creatinine

   d. Concomitant hepatic and renal failure

5. Yes; nausea, vomiting, fatigue, and scleral icterus indicate liver failure.

6. Both BUN and creatinine values may be increased falsely by dehydration, a condition that is probable in this patient. Creatinine clearance results are not affected as dramatically by dehydration.

7. Clearance is defined as the volume of plasma from which a measured amount of a substance can be completely eliminated into the urine per unit of time. The formula for calculating creatinine clearance is

$$\text{Clearance} = \frac{U \times V}{P}$$

where U equals the urine creatinine concentration, expressed in mg/dL; V equals the volume of urine collected, expressed in mL/min; and P equals the plasma concentration of creatinine, expressed in mg/dL. You may also adapt this calculation to correct for the patient's body surface area by including a comparison to a standard body surface area. The formula for this calculation is

$$\text{Clearance} = \frac{U \times V}{P} \times \frac{1.73}{\text{BSA}}$$

where 1.73 represents standard body surface area and BSA is found using the patient's height and weight from a nomogram.

Creatinine clearance results are reported in mL/min and are gender-specific.

8. Renal clearance tests provide important information about the effectiveness of the kidneys in performing their excretory functions. The use of clearance tests enables the evaluation of the kidneys' effectiveness in performing functions such as glomerular filtration or tubular secretion. Clearance tests are the best laboratory evaluations to detect mild to moderate diffuse glomerular damage and are generally performed to evaluate the glomerular filtration rate.

Study Questions B

1. Decreased renal function that improved as the patient was rehydrated and treated. This patient did not have normal creatinine clearance results on 7/31, even though the serum BUN and creatinine were approaching normal.

2. Any serum creatinine value above 2.0 mg/dL is considered abnormal, and when it rises above 10 mg/dL, it is considered a critical value. Mr. Roberts's serum creatinine increased from 7.2 mg/dL on 7/20 to 9.6 mg/dL on 7/21 and exceeded 10 mg/dL on 7/22, when it was 12.8 mg/dL. Serum creatinine peaked on 7/23 at 14.3 mg/dL.

3. The renal failure is secondary to acetaminophen overdose and is worsened by dehydration from the severe vomiting caused by the liver problem.

4. Acute renal failure occurs in less than 2 percent of all acetaminophen poisonings and 10 percent of severely poisoned patients. At therapeutic dosages, acetaminophen can be toxic to the kidneys in patients who are glutathione depleted (as a result of chronic alcohol ingestion, starvation, or fasting) or who take drugs that stimulate the P-450 microsomal oxidase enzymes (anticonvulsants). Acute renal failure due to acetaminophen manifests as acute tubular necrosis (ATN). ATN can occur alone or in combination with hepatic necrosis. The azotemia of acetaminophen toxicity is typically reversible, although it may worsen over 7 to 10 days before the recovery of renal function occurs. In severe overdoses, renal failure coincides with hepatic encephalopathy, and dialysis may be required.

5. a. The extremely high AST (16,960 IU/L) and ALT activities (10,680 IU/L)

    b. **Infections:** The most common infectious cause is viral hepatitis, particularly of HBV origin, with herpes simplex virus and Epstein-Barr virus also being frequently seen.

    Poisons, chemicals, or drugs: While there are many toxic substances that may produce fulminant hepatic failure, the three most common are ingestion of mushrooms of *Amanita* species, individual toxic responses to common antibiotics such as tetracycline, and intentional or accidental overdose of acetaminophen.

Hepatic ischemia: Heat stroke and prolonged impaired blood flow during surgery may be followed by fulminant hepatic failure. Budd-Chiari syndrome, thrombosis of the hepatic veins, will also result in this condition.

c. The acetaminophen had been consumed at least 48 h previous to his admission, and he had a history of vomiting during that time. Whatever amount of analgesic had been absorbed before this episode began had already been metabolized and excreted by the time of presentation.

6. Many of the coagulation factors are synthesized in the liver. When the liver fails, these coagulation factors are not made and/or released, and the patient is likely to have bleeding problems. FFP contains fresh coagulation factors, and vitamin K is necessary for the liver to synthesize these coagulation factors. The treatment was administered prophylactically to prevent bleeding.

7. a. Within several hours of ingestion, the patient develops nausea, vomiting, and hypotension. This initial phase may then subside and the patient will exhibit few symptoms, but over the next 24 to 48 h there appears clinical and laboratory evidence of progressive deterioration of liver function.

    b. Use of an antidote, either N-acetylcysteine or methionine, is appropriate for acute acetaminophen overdose. Either antidote enters into the metabolic pathways via glutathione mechanisms to preclude the formation of an epoxide derivative of acetaminophen that binds covalently to liver macromolecules, resulting in destruction of the liver cells.

    c. This treatment should be initiated within 12 h to be effective.

    d. Treatment of chronic acetaminophen poisoning is to support the liver and renal failure.

    e. The primary clinical effect of acetaminophen poisoning is hepatotoxicity, which occurs after ingestion of large single doses of acetaminophen or after ingestion of smaller doses in patients with a hepatic metabolism that is altered by drugs or concurrent medicalconditions.Hepatocellular damage is probably caused by accumulation of the toxic intermediate metabolite N-acetyl-p-benzoquinoneimine when hepatic glutathione stores are depleted.

    Moderate to heavy alcohol use potentiates the toxic effects of acetaminophen. Acute toxic effects on the liver are seen in long-term alcohol users who have ingested therapeutic doses of acetaminophen. Severe hepatotoxicity may occur after ingestion of as little as 4 g in 24 h.

8. No; acetaminophen and/or alcohol determinations on this patient would have been inappropriate considering the time of ingestion of these substances and the time of the patient's admission.

9. The laboratory played an integral part in the diagnosis, monitoring, and evaluation of treatment in this patient. The seriousness and instability of Mr. Roberts' condition required frequent monitoring of several analytes to properly evaluate his status.

CASE SUMMARY

PATIENT: WALTER ROBERTS

Mr. Roberts is a 39-year-old white male with no significant past medical history who presented with a 2-day history of severe nausea and vomiting. Physical examination showed him to be moderately jaundiced. The patient's blood pressure was 140/98, temperature 99°F, pulse 80 and regular, and respiration 30 and unlabored. His history is negative for medical or surgical illnesses, and he has had no blood transfusions or known exposure to hepatitis. He admits to being under extreme stress at his job. Further questioning reveals a 2-year history of chronic headaches and self-medication with extra-strength Tylenol, taking 4 to 10 per day regularly. In addition, alcohol consumption consists of three or four rum-and-Cokes routinely on weekday evenings and a higher intake on the weekends. Within the past 2 weeks, he has participated in a half-court basketball game without undue fatigue. He denies any recent myalgias or arthralgias and states that he was completely well until 48 h prior to admission.

After Mr. Roberts' admission laboratory results were reviewed, he was admitted to the ICU to determine the cause of his abnormal results. He received 2 units of fresh frozen plasma and 20 mg of vitamin K intravenously. Intense monitoring of the patient's physical and mental status was undertaken during the initial hospital days. The patient showed no deterioration in these regards.

Mr. Roberts' problems are twofold: he has both severe liver damage and poor renal function. Each of these situations calls for immediate and complete care and treatment.

The liver function studies are inconclusive as to the nature of the hepatitis. While the hepatitis profile rules out hepatitis A, B, and C, other causes of viral hepatitis are still an option. Hepatitis E and G and other non-A, non-E hepatitis viruses are unlikely considering his travel and social history, but other hepatotoxic viruses such as cytomegalovirus or Epstein-Barr virus cannot be ruled out. The hepatotoxic effects of acetaminophen are widely documented, although most cases are of acute poisoning, not chronic abuse. Because of the severe nature of the liver insult and the high degree of hepatocellular necrosis, consultation with a liver transplant team was obtained even though the liver/spleen scan showed fairly good liver function. Daily serial laboratory tests for liver functions showed a steady decrease in all liver parameters after admission.

The urine output was quite small on admission, and repeated renal parameters revealed that the BUN and creatinine were rapidly increasing, resulting in consultation with the nephrology service. On the third hospital day, the patient was transferred from the ICU to a regular floor, where renal dialysis was initiated. After dialysis, urine output increased and BUN and creatinine began a return to normal.

After a hospital stay of 14 days, Mr. Roberts was discharged in much improved condition, to be followed as an outpatient with regard to his renal function, his liver function, and the cause of his recurrent headaches. The patient refused to return for reevaluation of either renal or liver status.

Patients who have alcohol-acetaminophen syndrome have a worse prognosis than patients with only acetaminophen overdose, even if the former have ingested a lower dose of acetaminophen. Overall mortality in alcohol-acetaminophen syndrome is 18 to 19 percent. When acute liver failure develops, the mortality rate exceeds 75 percent. If the patient is successfully supported through the liver failure, a return to normal hepatic function is expected within 3 months.

This patient's renal failure was corrected with hydration and renal dialysis, with no lasting damage to the kidneys.

ANSWERS TO LEARNING ACTIVITIES

PATIENT: AARON SHAPELY

Study Questions A

1. *Clinical Symptoms:* Productive cough, fever, night sweats, unexplained weight loss

   Background History: Chronic hepatitis B, intermittent oral herpes, HIV positive

2. *Blood culture × 3; *sputum bacterial, *AFB, *fungal cultures; *lung tissue culture for bacteria, *AFB, *fungi; *smear for *Pneumocystis carinii*

   * = Tests that correlate with presenting symptoms

4. a. Blood cultures showed aerobic growth after 4 days of incubation. Sputum cultures grew the same organism isolated from the blood cultures. The lymphocyte profile showed a greatly decreased CD4/CD8 ratio. The absolute CD4 count was 98 (normal count is >500).

   b. These results indicate that the patient is in the late stages of AIDS. His presenting symptoms are typical for AIDS patients.

5. The skin biopsy showed Kaposi sarcoma, an indicator for AIDS. A request to examine tissue samples for *P. carinii* was made.

Study Questions B

1. Gram-positive non-spore-forming rods were isolated from the blood cultures incubated under an aerobic environment. For subcultures on blood agar and chocolate agar plates, nonhemolytic colonies grew after 24 h of incubation. The organisms were catalase positive. The isolate was reported as *Corynebacterium jeikeium*. Antimicrobial susceptibility showed an extremely resistant organism. However, further investigation revealed that the isolate had been misidentified. The correct identification of the organism was *Rhodococcus equi*.

2. a. On Gram-stained smears, *R. equi* appears as gram-positive non-spore-forming rods in various lengths and forms and has been described as resembling members of the genus *Corynebacterium*; hence, it was formerly known as *Corynebacterium equi*. Because of the "diphtheroid" morphologic form of the organism, *R. equi* may be regarded as a skin contaminant, particularly when it was isolated from blood cultures, respiratory secretions, and other clinical samples obtained using invasive procedures.

   b. Morphologic differentiation of *R. equi* from corynebacteria may be made by comparing its microscopic morphology on smears made directly from clinical samples or from solid medium with the morphology that is observed in smears prepared from broth medium. When smears are made from a solid medium or a clinical sample, *R. equi* appears as coccoid or coccobacillary, whereas in a liquid or broth medium, these organisms form long, curly, sometimes branching filamentous rods. Biochemically, *R. equi* is nonmotile and produces catalase like most corynebacteria. Differentiation from other gram-positive non-spore-forming rods may be accomplished based on its characteristic colonial morphology, a salmon pink coloration that develops as the culture ages, and its inability to ferment carbohydrates or liquefy gelatin.

3. *C. jeikeium*, formerly *Corynebacterium JK*, has become a clinically significant isolate when it is found in blood and other normally sterile body fluids of patients who are immunocompromised. Although this bacterial species is not usually found in the normal skin flora of healthy individuals in the community, it is not uncommon to encounter this organism in the skin flora of hospitalized patients. This organism may cause serious nosocomial infections, such as endocarditis, infections of the CSF shunts, osteomyelitis, and pneumonia.

   C. jeikeium has been isolated from patients with hematologic disorders, those receiving chemotherapy, bone marrow transplant recipients, and patients with AIDS. Factors that predispose patients to *C. jeikeium* infections include instrumentation, such as an indwelling catheter, and prosthetic valve placement, as well as prolonged hospitalization and severe neutropenia. A key factor in the significance of *C. jeikeium* is its resistance to multiple antimicrobials.

R. equi is an organism known to be pathogenic for a variety of animals, including horses, swine, and cattle. Found in the gastrointestinal tract of herbivores, this organism is widely distributed in the environment, particularly in soil where animals graze. It is therefore believed to be acquired by inhalation and causes chronic granulomatous pneumonia and lung abscesses in these animals. Until recently, infections in humans have been rare, with the majority occurring in immunocompromised patients, primarily those with lymphoma and neoplastic disease. During recent years, these organisms have occurred in a variety of pulmonary infections, such as pneumonia and lung abscess, in AIDS patients.

Pulmonary clearance of *R. equi* requires functional T lymphocytes, particularly the T4 helper cells (CD4+ fraction). This is the same fraction that is affected in AIDS, which explains why this organism is especially virulent in these patients. The mortality rate for AIDS patients infected by *R. equi* is 25 percent.

4. *Pneumocystis carinii* pneumonia (PCP) remains the most common life-threatening opportunistic infection encountered in patients with HIV. Until recently, when aggressive PCP prophylaxis and multiple drug combinations for treatment of HIV infection appeared, PCP was the CDC's defined index diagnosis in patients with HIV disease. With new treatment and wider use of prophylaxis during recent years, the incidence of AIDS patients diagnosed with PCP prior to death has decreased to 42.3 percent from 85 percent early in the epidemic. Finally, it has been shown that patients who have CD4 counts less than 200 cells per microliter and who are not receiving prophylaxis are most likely to acquire PCP.

CASE SUMMARY

PATIENT: AARON SHAPELY

A 53-year-old white male patient was admitted to the clinic for an annual physical. The patient's symptoms, on admission, included a productive cough, fever, night sweats, and unexplained weight loss. The patient had previously been diagnosed as HIV positive. He also had a history of chronic hepatitis B and intermittent oral herpes. The patient had seen his personal physician, been diagnosed with bronchitis, and been unsuccessfully treated with Augmentin.

At the physical examination, the patient presented with skin discolorations, which were biopsied. His lung x-rays revealed a large upper lobe infiltrate with cavitation formation. The patient was admitted to the hospital, and lung tissue biopsies, skin biopsies, blood, and sputum were all evaluated.

The skin biopsies proved to be positive for Kaposi sarcoma. His lymphocyte profile revealed that his CD4/CD8 ratio was greatly decreased to 0.08 (normal is 1.5–2.0). His absolute CD4 count was 98 (normal is >5000). The blood, sputum, and biopsy materials were sent to microbiology for culture. After 4 days, the aerobic blood culture grew a gram-positive rod (diphtheroid). No growth occurred in the anaerobic bottle. Overnight cultures grown on blood agar and chocolate agar revealed a tiny, nonhemolytic, catalase-positive organism. The organism was multiply resistant to cephalothin, clindamycin, nitrofuratoin, penicillin, tetracycline, and trimethoprim-sulfamethoxazole, and sensitive to erythromycin, ofloxacin, and vancomycin.

Because of the multiple-resistance pattern, the organism was originally reported as *Corynebacterium JK*. The physician questioned the results, whereupon the lab personnel reexamined the original plates (now over 48 h old). The colonies had begun to turn a pinkish salmon color and were mucoid in consistency. An acid-fast stain showed the organism to be partially acid-fast. GLC analysis of the methyl fatty acid esters was consistent with *Rhodococcus equi*. A second blood culture drawn 3 days after the first was submitted grew *R. equi*. The sputum also grew *R. equi*. The lung biopsy was negative for bacterial pathogens; mycobacteria still pending; no *Pneumocystis carinii* or other fungi (*Cryptococcus neoformans*, any dimorphic fungi, *Aspergillus*) were recovered.

The final diagnosis was that the patient was suffering from a rhodococcal lung infection exacerbated by his advanced stage of AIDS. He was treated by IV with vancomycin, erythromycin, ofloxacin, and rifampin. The fever subsided, and no additional isolates were recovered from the blood. The patient was given long-term antimicrobial therapy to suppress the organism and released from the hospital.

ANSWERS TO LEARNING ACTIVITIES

PATIENT: JASON STEWART

Study Questions A

1. *Clinical Symptoms:* Dysphasia

    Background History: No background history known or noted in the medical records

2. *CBC

    * = Tests that correlate with presenting symptoms

4. a. High white blood cell count was observed, with absolute lymphocytosis.

    b. The peripheral blood smears basically have the hallmark signs of chronic lymphocytic leukemia (CCL) in that they show a predominance of small, mature lymphocytes to the virtual exclusion of all other types of WBCs. Additionally, a high percentage of smudge cells are observed. Smudge cells result from the smear preparation of a person with CLL and are considered to be a hallmark of the disease. Because there were no blasts observed on the blood smears or noted on the CBC results, acute lymphocytic and myelogenous leukemias can be eliminated. Since no neutrophils or neutrophil precursors were noted on the smears, a diagnosis of chronic myelogenous leukemia is not indicated. Thus, the CBC results and blood smears indicate that this person is suffering from CLL.

5. The flow cytometry results provide a further diagnosis of CLL. The malignant cells of each type of leukemia show a characteristic pattern of CD antigen expression. The CD marker expression in this patient is consistent will B-cell CLL. The positivity for both CD19 and CD5 basically rules out all other leukemias in that CLL is the only type that expresses both of these markers. Although not discussed earlier, the flow cytometry results rule out the possibility of a lymphoma, as no lymphomas express the group of CD markers seen with this patient.

A diagnosis of CLL must meet the following criteria:

(1) Absolute lymphocyte count in the peripheral blood >10,000, with the majority appearing to be small lymphocytes. (2) B-cell phenotype of circulating lymphocytes.

Both of these criteria are met based on the REAL classification, although the WHO 2001 classification may provide a more precise delineation.

6. Chronic lymphocytic leukemia (CCL)

7. a. Using the Rai Clinical Staging System for CLL, the patient is in Stage 0. Stage 0 is characterized by lymphocytosis in the blood and bone marrow with no indications of pancytopenia or organ enlargement. As the lymphocytes continue to proliferate in a person with CLL, they literally push out all other types of cells from the marrow. The patient often suffers from symptoms of pancytopenia, such as anemia or infections. In addition, the malignant cells often infiltrate various tissues of the body, such as the liver, spleen, or lymph nodes. The physical examination of the patient showed no signs of pancytopenia or organ enlargement. A higher Rai classification would indicate that the disease was progressing more aggressively.

b. In patients with Rai Stage 0 CLL, no treatment is initiated. Instead, the patient will return to the hospital for a physical exam along with a CBC and blood smear examination. Based on the results, the patient may remain at Rai Stage 0 or progress to a higher level. Rai Stage 1 involves the initiation of chemotherapy. Some 50 percent of patients diagnosed with CLL are alive 5 years after diagnosis. Some 30 percent are alive 10 years after diagnosis.

CASE SUMMARY

PATIENT: JASON STEWART

The patient is a 72-year-old male who presented to the Health Clinic complaining of dysphasia. His physical examination showed no signs of leukemia, such as fever, fatigue, weight loss, or any organ enlargement. During the blood work-up for the patient, a high white blood cell count was observed, with absolute lymphocytosis. Based on the initial findings, a diagnosis of leukemia was made, and the patient was referred for further work-up and laboratory studies.

The peripheral blood smears showed a predominance of small, mature lymphocytes with a high number of smudge cells. Flow cytometric analysis demonstrated that the lymphocytes co-expressed CD19, CD5, and CD23, in addition to other B-cell markers. This nearly defines CLL.

A diagnosis of chronic lymphocytic leukemia was made based on the morphologic features observed on the peripheral smears; they showed a predominance of small, mature lymphocytes to the virtual exclusion of all other types of WBCs. In addition, a high percentage of smudge cells was observed. The absence of blasts on the blood smears ruled out an acute stage, while the absence of neutrophils or neutrophil precursors noted on the smears meant that a diagnosis of chronic myelogenous leukemia was not indicated. The CBC results, blood smears, and flow cytometry indicated that this person was suffering from CLL.

The overall prognosis for this patient is good. Using the Rai Clinical Staging System for CLL, the patient is in Stage 0. Stage 0 is characterized by lymphocytosis in the blood and bone marrow, with no indications of pancytopenia or organ enlargement. As the lymphocytes continue to proliferate in a person with CLL, they literally push out all other types of cells from the marrow. A patient often suffers from symptoms of pancytopenia, such as anemia or infections. In addition, the malignant cells often infiltrate various tissues of the body, such as the liver, spleen, or lymph nodes. The physical examination of the patient showed no signs of pancytopenia or organ enlargement. A higher Rai classification would indicate that the disease was progressing more aggressively.

In patients with Rai Stage 0 CLL, no treatment is initiated. Instead, the patient will return to the hospital for a physical examination along with a CBC and blood smear examination. Based on the results, the patient may remain at Rai Stage 0 or progress to a higher level. Rai Stage 1 involves the initiation of chemotherapy. Some 50 percent of patients diagnosed with CLL live for 5 years after the diagnosis is made, while 30 percent live for 10 years after the diagnosis.

PATIENT: IRMA VAN HEUSEN

Study Questions A

1. *Clinical Symptoms:* Shortness of breath, nausea and vomiting, fever, chills, rigor

    Background History: Pacemaker insertion 10 days prior

2. *Glucose, *BUN, *electrolytes, *urinalysis, *CBC, *cardiac enzymes, *blood cultures × 2

    * = Tests that correlate with presenting symptoms

4. a. Glucose, BUN, and electrolytes were within the reference range. Cardiac enzymes also showed within normal limits, which ruled out cardiac infarct.

    The CBC showed leukocytosis. The differential count showed neutrophilia with shift to the left and toxic granulations.

    b. Toxic granulation is usually associated with bacterial infection and when present provides a clue to the differential diagnosis of leukocytosis when leukemia is also being considered as a possible diagnosis. Other toxic changes that may be present are the appearance of Döhle bodies and vacuoles. The patient presented with fever, chills, and rigor. Fever, although it may be provoked by a variety of stimuli, is most often caused by bacteria and their endotoxins, viruses, and other types of microorganisms. Fever may also occur during an inflammatory reaction in tissues and blood vessels or as a result of the destruction of tissues through events such as trauma. The patient's symptoms correlate with the morphologic indicators of an infection.

5. The blood culture results will be significant.

Study Questions B

1. The blood culture results showed two different organisms. Blood culture set 1 was first reported to grow viridans streptococci; this was later corrected to *Leuconostoc* species. Enterococci were reported on the second set of blood cultures.

2. The patient had a history of pacemaker insertion prior to presenting with clinical symptoms. This invasive procedure may have facilitated the entry of the organisms into the bloodstream when the first line of defense, the skin, was compromised.

3. The microscopic and colonial morphology of *Leuconostoc* can be easily mistaken for similar-looking or closely related species. Some of these species are normal skin colonizers; hence, the isolate may be interpreted as a skin contaminant and therefore clinically insignificant unless a full investigation is performed.

CASE SUMMARY

PATIENT: IRMA VAN HEUSEN

This case involved a 64-year-old white female who was admitted to the hospital with primary complaints of shortness of breath, nausea, vomiting, rigor, and chills. Her clinical history included pacemaker insertion 10 days prior to admission. Further physical examination revealed atrial fibrillation and mitral valve regurgitation. Laboratory findings on admission showed cardiac enzymes within normal ranges, which ruled out myocardial infarct. Other admitting laboratory findings were unremarkable and were within normal ranges. The patient was admitted to the Coronary Care Unit for observation. Two sets of blood cultures were obtained. After 48 h of incubation, all blood cultures showed growth. On smear examination, gram-positive cocci were observed.

At 18 to 24 h, subculture plates from the blood cultures grew catalase-negative gram-positive cocci. Blood culture set 1 grew alpha-hemolytic, vancomycin-resistant gram-positive cocci, later identified as *Leuconostoc*. Set 2 grew nonhemolytic, catalase-negative gram-positive cocci identified as *Enterococcus* species. The patient was placed on gentamicin and penicillin for 4 weeks and was subsequently released from the hospital. Follow-up blood cultures were negative.

ANSWERS TO LEARNING ACTIVITIES

PATIENT: BEATRICE WEST

Study Questions A

1. *Clinical Symptoms:* Fever, malaise, abdominal pain

   Background History: No background history noted

2. Based on Ms. West's laboratory findings, she was diagnosed with acute lymphocytic anemia, which predisposed her to her infection.

3. *CBC, *blood cultures, *glucose, *BUN, *electrolytes

   * = Tests that correlate with presenting symptoms

5. a. Ms. West's CBC showed a white blood cell count of 19,500/mm³ with 54 percent blasts. Bone marrow aspirate provided a diagnosis of acute lymphocytic leukemia.

b. With this diagnosis, she became immunocompromised and susceptible to infectious diseases.

6. Results of the blood cultures will be important. Follow up or repeat WBC.

Study Questions B

1. *Trichosporon beigelii* was isolated from the skin biopsy and blood cultures. The blood cultures also yielded *Candida tropicalis*.

2. Ms. West was diagnosed with acute lymphocytic leukemia, a hematologic disorder that made her predisposed to infections such as that caused by *T. beigelii*. Although this organism can be found as a normal skin inhabitant in normal healthy individuals, in an immunocompromised person such as Ms. West, it has been reported to cause a serious, life-threatening disseminated form of infection. The disease may present in an acute form, with manifestations such as nodular skin lesions, general malaise, fever, and pulmonary infiltrates, the clinical presentations shown by the patient.

3. Although *Trichosporon* species are morphologically distinct from *Candida* species in the structures they produce, such as arthroconidia and blastoconidia, and the assimilation patterns they show, initial testing with latex agglutination test for cyrptococcal antigen can be misleading. Sera from patients with dissiminated *T. beigelii* infections have shown positive reactions to the latex agglutination test. Nevertheless, the results of the test, although misleading, provide an initial diagnosis of fungemia, which directs the institution of appropriate therapy.

Patients with disseminated trichosporonosis have a serious prognosis despite aggressive antifungal therapy; nearly 75 percent yield to their infection. Although amphotericin B is active against many fungal infections, it has limited activity against *Trichosporon* species.

CASE SUMMARY

PATIENT: BEATRICE WEST

The patient was a 55-year-old female who presented with fever, malaise, and mild abdominal pain. On admission, her white blood cell count was 19,500/mm^3 with 54 percent blast cells found in the peripheral smear differential count. Bone marrow aspirate gave a diagnosis of acute lymphocytic leukemia. Three sets of blood cultures were drawn. On 4/5, she had a temperature spike. She was placed on empiric therapy with broad-spectrum antibiotics. She also began induction chemotherapy. She became afebrile, but her white blood cell count fell to <500 cells/mm^3.

The patient also became disoriented and developed a reddish nodular rash on her trunk and extremities. She also developed bilateral interstitial pulmonary infiltrates and hypoxemia. She then required mechanical ventilation.

Within 48 h of incubation, the blood cultures grew yeasts, and her antimicrobial regimen was changed to vancomycin, ticarcillin, erythromycin, and gentamicin. Amphotericin B therapy was also initiated. Her granulocytes at this time remained at 250 cells/mm^3. A serum latex agglutination test for cryptococcal antigen was positive at a titer of 1:8.

Over the next 36 h, she became unstable and suffered cardiac arrest, from which she could not be resuscitated. Biopsy of a lesion revealed arthroconidia, blastoconidia, and pseudohyphae. These structures were consistent with *Trichosporon beigelii*. Cultures of the skin biopsy grew *T. beigelii*, and blood culture isolates were identified as *Candida tropicalis* and *T. beigelii*.

ANSWERS TO LEARNING ACTIVITIES

PATIENT: LENA WILSON

Study Questions A

1. *Clinical Symptoms:* Shortness of breath, fatigue, muscle pain/back pain

   Background History: Previously diagnosed with AML M4, chemotherapy and bone marrow transplant, previous BM biopsy showed remission

2. *CBC, total bilirubin type and cross-match

   * = Tests that correlate with presenting symptoms

4. a. Abnormally low RBC, Hgb, and Hct combined with normal MCH, MCHC, MCV, and RDW indicate a quantitative red cell deficiency.

   b. Her shortness of breath and fatigue can be attributed to her abnormally low hemoglobin and hematocrit. The presence of blasts (16 percent) with Auer rods and thrombocytopenia combined with anemia are characteristic features of her diagnosed condition.

5. Flow cytometry studies determined whether the current condition was a relapse or a different type of disorder. Bone marrow biopsy and aspiration determined the status of the bone marrow, which revealed a marked decrease in red blood cell precursors and that a large proportion of the cells were immature granulocytes, with 10 to 15 percent blasts.

   Normal bilirubin levels and no evidence of splenomegaly discounted the likelihood of increased red blood cell destruction as a cause of her anemia.

Study Questions B

1. a. Based on the CBC, an initial diagnosis of anemia and thrombocytopenia was made. Causes of anemia and thrombocytopenia can be categorized as increased destruction or decreased production. The decrease in multiple cell lines indicated bone marrow involvement. The presence

of blasts in the peripheral blood also indicated bone marrow involvement. Bone marrow abnormalities are indicative of decreased production. Normal bilirubin levels and no evidence of splenomegaly discounted the likelihood of increased destruction as a cause.

b. The presence of blasts in the peripheral blood confirmed bone marrow involvement. The presence of Auer rods in a few of the blasts indicated a myeloid cell lineage.

c. Bone marrow abnormalities are indicative of decreased production. With decreased production as the likely cause of the anemia and thrombocytopenia, it was necessary to confirm bone marrow involvement by observation of the bone marrow biopsy. Observation under low power revealed 95 percent cellularity, whereas 50 percent cellularity would be expected in a person this age. Significant fibrosis was also noted. Observation under high power revealed a marked decrease in red cell precursors and decreased megakaryocytes. A large proportion of cells were immature granulocytes, with 10 to 15 percent blasts.

The presence of blasts in the peripheral blood and bone marrow indicated an acute leukemia disorder. In an adult patient, the majority of cases are of myeloid origin. This is supported by the presence of Auer rods in the blasts and the presence of granulocytic precursors in the bone marrow. These findings are sufficient for a diagnosis of acute myelogenous leukemia.

2. In order to determine if this was a relapse of the previously diagnosed disease, flow cytometry was conducted. The results indicated that the blasts were of myeloid descent, but were negative for monocytic markers. This is a change from the original diagnosis.

From examination of the patient's peripheral blood, bone marrow, and flow cytometry, the final diagnosis was determined as a relapse of acute myeloid leukemia.

CASE SUMMARY

PATIENT: LENA WILSON

The patient is a 38-year-old Caucasian female who had been previously diagnosed with AML M4 15 months prior. She presented with shortness of breath, muscle ache, and fatigue. She had received treatment for her leukemia that included chemotherapeutic drugs and a bone marrow transplant. A bone marrow biopsy 10 months prior to this visit indicated complete remission. On this present admission, complete blood count results showed an abnormally low RBC, Hgb, and Hct combined with normal MCH, MCHC, MCV, and RDW, an indication of a quantitative red cell deficiency. Decreased platelets along with the low red cell count is also an indication of bone marrow involvement.

The peripheral blood showed blasts present; Auer rods in a few of the blasts point toward a myeloid cell lineage. The presence of blasts in the peripheral blood also indicated that the bone marrow was involved.

Based on the CBC, an initial diagnosis of anemia and thrombocytopenia was made. Causes of anemia and thrombocytopenia can be categorized as either increased destruction or decreased production of these cellular components. Generally, the decrease in multiple cell lines indicates bone marrow involvement. Bone marrow abnormalities are indicative of decreased production. Normal bilirubin levels and no evidence of splenomegaly discounted the likelihood of increased destruction as a cause.

With decreased production as the likely cause of the anemia and thrombocytopenia, it was necessary to confirm bone marrow involvement by observing a bone marrow biopsy.

Observation of the bone marrow biopsy under low power revealed 95 percent cellularity, whereas 50 percent cellularity would be expected in a person this age. Significant fibrosis was also noted. Observation under high power revealed a marked decrease in red cell precursors and decreased megakaryocytes. The large proportion of cells were immature granulocytes, with 10 to 15 percent blasts.

The presence of blasts in the peripheral blood and bone marrow indicated an acute leukemia disorder. In an adult patient, the majority of cases are of myeloid origin. This is supported by the presence of Auer rods in the blasts and the presence of granulocytic precursors in the bone marrow. These findings are sufficient for a diagnosis of acute myelogenous leukemia. In order to determine if this was a relapse of the previously diagnosed disease, flow cytometry was conducted. The results indicated that the blasts were of myeloid descent, but were negative for monocytic markers. This is a change from the original diagnosis.

After a close examination of the patient's peripheral blood, bone marrow, and flow cytometry, the final diagnosis is a relapse of acute myeloid leukemia with a slightly different presentation from that of the original disease.

ANSWERS TO LEARNING ACTIVITIES

PATIENT: DANNON WISE

Study Questions A

1. *Clinical Symptoms*: Fever, anorexia, lethargy, dehydration

   Background History: Osteomyelitis, alcohol abuse, renal disease/failure, diabetes

2. *CBC, *glucose, *electrolytes, *urinalysis, *BUN, *CSF analysis, *blood cultures, *CSF cultures, *urine culture

   * = Tests that correlate with presenting symptoms

4. Glucose, BUN, and electrolytes were all within the reference ranges. Urinalysis results showed protein in her urine, and a microscopic exam showed an abnormal number of leukocytes, red blood cells, and numerous bacteria indicating a possible urinary tract infection. The WBC count was elevated and was outside the acceptable reference range, indicating leukocytosis. The differential count shows neutrophilia, indicative of infection.

5. The CSF analysis showed an increased number of WBCs, decreased glucose concentration, and increased protein. Culture results of the CSF, blood, and urine should also be considered.

Study Questions B

1. Microbiology culture results produced growth of a bacterial species identified as *Listeria monocytogenes*. Blood cultures grew the same organisms. *Escherichia coli*, colony count >100,000 CFU/mL, was isolated from the urine.

2. *L. monocytogenes* is usually acquired by ingesting contaminated food. Unlike other food-borne pathogens, however, the disease manifests as a systemic disease such as bacteremia or meningitis rather than as a diarrheal illness.

3. Ms. Wise has numerous risk factors that may have contributed to her illness. These include her age and the presence of chronic illness, such as diabetes and renal disease. Alcohol abuse and heavy smoking are also considered to be health risk factors. *L. monocytogenes* has been reported to be the third most frequent cause of community-acquired bacterial meningitis in adults. In particular, immunocompromised individuals such as those with hematologic malignancies, those with AIDS, recipients of organ transplantation, and those receiving corticosteroid therapy are at highest risk for the disease.

4. As in infections caused by other bacterial species, early in the infection, the CSF in listeriosis may appear normal. Unlike other forms of meningitis, however, listeria meningitis/meningoencephalitis rarely elicits a high white blood cell count or a high concentration of protein (>200 mg/dL) in the CSF. In addition, the organisms are found only in approximately 40 percent of Gram-stained smears. Moreover, the microscopic characteristics of *L. monocytogenes* are variable and difficult to assess, showing pleomorphism and often resembling diphtheroids and certain streptococcal species. Hence, direct Gram-stained smear of the CSF does not provide helpful information either, unlike the situation in other bacterial meningitis infections, where the etiologic agent may be readily revealed by the bacterial microscopic morphology.

CASE SUMMARY

PATIENT: DANNON WISE

An 79-year-old female from a nursing home presented with confusion and refusal to eat and drink. On examination, she showed signs of a mild pneumonia. The patient was also febrile and showed signs of lethargy. The patient's past history revealed osteomyelitis of the foot, renal disease, heart failure, diverticulitis, and diabetes. She also had a history of alcohol abuse and heavy smoking.

Gram-stained smear from anaerobic blood culture showed gram-positive bacilli, and the culture grew out small, smooth, translucent colonies with a narrow zone of beta hemolysis. The organism was identified as *Listeria monocytogenes*. The CSF yielded similar results. The origin of sepsis was never clearly defined, but possibilities included contamination of diverticulitis, since the organism is sometimes found in human stool.

Treatment was started with ampicillin intravenously. The physician later altered treatment to a combination of ampicillin and penicillin. Gentamicin was later added to the regimen. The infection was resolved eventually, and the patient was discharged to the nursing home, where she continued to receive treatment.

► INDEX